VAGUS NERVE

Freedom From Anxiety, Trauma and Depression Through Polyvagal Theory

By

Bryan Miller

Copyright 2019

COPYRIGHT PAGE

This document is geared towards providing exact and reliable information with regards to the topic and issue covered. The publication is sold with the idea that the publisher is not required to render accounting, officially permitted, or otherwise, qualified services. If advice is necessary, legal or professional, a practiced individual in the profession should be ordered.

From a Declaration of Principles which was accepted and approved equally by a Committee of the American Bar Association and a Committee of Publishers and Associations.

In no way is it legal to reproduce, duplicate, or transmit any part of this document in either electronic means or in printed format. Recording of this publication is strictly prohibited and any storage of this document is not allowed unless with written permission from the publisher. All rights reserved.

The information provided herein is stated to be truthful and consistent, in that any liability, in terms of inattention or otherwise, by any usage or abuse of any policies, processes, or directions contained within is the solitary and utter responsibility of the recipient reader. Under no circumstances will any legal responsibility or blame be held against the publisher for any reparation, damages, or monetary loss due to the information herein, either directly or indirectly.

Respective authors own all copyrights not held by the publisher.

The information herein is offered for informational purposes solely, and is universal as so. The presentation of the information is without contract or any type of guarantee assurance.

The trademarks that are used are without any consent, and the publication of the trademark is without permission or backing by the trademark owner. All trademarks and brands within this book are for clarifying purposes only and are the owned by the owners themselves, not affiliated with this document.

Table of Contents

Contents

<u>INTRODUCTION</u>

The Vagus Nerve is the longest-running cranial nerve in your body. It is one of ten combined cranial nerves and runs from the stem of your mind right down. It is one of the most fundamental pieces of the body that the vast majority never knew was imperative to our prosperity as of not long ago. The Vagus Nerve, in any case, is not necessary. "Vagus" actually means "wandering" in Latin, and the Vagus Nerve satisfies its name. As the longest and generally complicated of all the cranial nerves, it begins at the stem of the mind, behind the ears before it wanders down the sides of the neck, through the chest, and in the long run finishes in the stomach area connecting the cerebrum to the heart, lungs, throat, and gut. This nerve must capacity appropriately with the goal for us to be robust, feel great inwardly, and connect emphatically with family, companions, and others. At the point when the ventral part of the vagus nerve and the related four cranial nerves work appropriately, individuals and different well-evolved creatures appreciate the alluring condition of social engagement. To be socially drawn in, we have to have a sense of security, with no compelling reason to survive or stay away from any outside danger by battling or escaping; we likewise should be physically robust. At the point when we are socially connected with, we don't have to do anything, or to transform anything; we can bear to be immobilized unafraid (loose). We can keep up an energetic tone without being fell or excessively excited.

CHAPTER ONE

UNDERSTANDING THE POLYVAGAL THEORY

The Polyvagal Theory: New Experiences into Versatile Responses of The Autonomic Nervous System

The polyvagal theory depicts an autonomic nervous system that is impacted by the focal nervous system, touchy to afferent impacts, described by a versatile reactivity reliant on the phylogeny of the neural circuits, and intuitive with source cores in the brainstem controlling the striated muscles of the face and head. The theory is subject to collected information portraying the phylogenetic advances in the vertebrate autonomic nervous system. Its particular spotlight is on the phylogenetic move among reptiles and vertebrates that brought about explicit changes to the vagal pathways controlling the heart. As the source cores of the essential vagal efferent pathways directing the heart moved from the dorsal engine core of the vagus in reptiles to the core ambiguous in warm-blooded creatures, a face–heart connection advanced with new properties of a social engagement system that would empower social associations to control instinctive state.

The polyvagal theory suggests that the advancement of the mammalian autonomic nervous system gives the neurophysiological substrates to versatile conduct methodologies. It further indicates that the physiological state confines the scope of conduct and mental experience. The theory connects the development of the autonomic nervous system to full of feeling experience, passionate demeanor, facial signals, vocal correspondence, and unexpected social conduct. Thusly, the theory gives a conceivable clarification to the detailed covariation between atypical autonomic guidelines (e.g., diminished vagal and expanded sympathetic impacts to the heart)

17

and mental and conduct issues that include troubles in managing suitable social, enthusiastic, and correspondence practices.

The polyvagal theory gives a few bits of knowledge into the versatile idea of a physiological state. Initially, the theory stresses that physiological states bolster various classes of conduct. For instance, a physiological state portrayed by a vagal withdrawal would bolster the activation practices of fight and flight. Interestingly, a physiological state characterized by the expanded vagal impact on the heart (using myelinated vagal pathways starting in the core ambiguous) would bolster unconstrained social engagement practices. Second, the theory accentuates the arrangement of an integrated social engagement system through useful and auxiliary connections between neural control of the striated muscles of the face and the smooth muscles of the viscera. Third, the polyvagal theory proposes an instrument—neuroception—to trigger or to repress guard techniques.

Picturing brain science can be something like picturing a typhoon. Although we can envision terrible climate, it is hard to envision changing that climate. In any case, Stephen Porges' polyvagal theory gives counsellors a valuable image of the nervous system that can direct us in our push to help customers. Porges' polyvagal theory created out of his tests with the vagus nerve. The vagus nerve serves the parasympathetic nervous system, which is the quieting part of our nervous system mechanics. The parasympathetic piece of the autonomic nervous system adjusts the sympathetic dynamic part, yet in substantially more nuanced ways than we comprehended before polyvagal theory.

Before polyvagal theory, our nervous system was imagined as a two-section opposing system, with more actuation flagging not so much quieting but rather more quieting flagging less initiation. The polyvagal theory distinguishes a third kind of nervous system reaction that Porges calls the social commitment system, a fun-loving blend of initiation and quieting that works out of novel nerve impact. The social engagement system helps us explore relationships. Helping our customers move into the utilization of their social commitment system enables them to turn out to be increasingly adaptable in their adapting styles.

The two different pieces of our nervous system capacity to help us oversee hazardous circumstances. Most counsellors are now acquainted with the two barrier instruments activated by these two pieces of the nervous system: sympathetic battle or-flight and parasympathetic shutdown, some of the time called freeze-or-black out. Utilization of our social commitment system, then again, requires a feeling of wellbeing. Polyvagal theory helps us comprehend that the two branches of the vagus nerve quiet the body; however, they do as such in various manners. Shutdown, or freeze-or-swoon, happens through the dorsal branch of the vagus nerve. This response can feel like the exhausted muscles and unsteadiness of terrible influenza. At the point when the dorsal vagal nerve closes down the body, it can move us into idleness or separation. Notwithstanding influencing the heart and lungs, the dorsal branch affects body working underneath the stomach and is engaged with stomach related problems.

The ventral branch of the vagal nerve influences body working over the stomach. This is the branch that serves the social commitment system. The ventral vagal nerve hoses the body's routinely dynamic state. Picture controlling a steed as you ride it back to the stable. You would keep on pulling back on and discharge the reins in nuanced approaches to guarantee that the steed keeps up a fitting velocity. Similarly, the ventral vagal nerve permits initiation in a nuanced way, in this way offering an unexpected quality in comparison to sympathetic actuation. Ventral vagal discharge into action takes milliseconds, while sympathetic initiation takes seconds and includes different substance responses that are much the same as losing the steed's reins. Also, when the battle or-flight synthetic reactions have started, it can take our bodies 10–20 minutes to come back to our pre-battle/pre-flight state. Ventral vagal discharge into action doesn't include these sorts of substance responses. In this way, we can make brisk changes among initiation and quieting, like what we can do when we utilize the reins to control the pony.

If you go to a pooch park, you will see certain mutts that are apprehensive. They show battle or-flight practices. Different pooches will flag a desire to play. This flagging frequently takes the structure that we people enlisted for the descending confronting hound present in yoga. At the point when a canine gives this sign, it signals a degree of excitement that can be serious. In any case, this perky vitality has an altogether different soul than the power of battle or-flight practices. This lively soul portrays the social commitment system. At the point when we experience our condition as protected, we work from our social commitment system.

THE POLYVAGAL PERSPECTIVE

The Polyvagal Theory presented another perspective of view relating autonomic capacity to conduct that incorporated a valuation for autonomic nervous system as a "system," the recognizable proof of neural circuits associated with the guideline of autonomic state, and a translation of autonomic reactivity as versatile inside the setting of the phylogeny of the vertebrate autonomic nervous system. The paper has two destinations: First, to give an express explanation of the theory; and second, to present the highlights of a polyvagal viewpoint. The polyvagal point of view accentuates how an understanding of neurophysiological systems and phylogenetic moves in a neural guideline, prompts various inquiries, ideal models, clarifications, and ends concerning autonomic capacity in biobehavioral forms than fringe models. Premier, the polyvagal point of view underlines the significance of phylogenetic changes in the neural structures directing the autonomic nervous system and how these phylogenetic movements give bits of knowledge into the versatile capacity and the neural guideline of the two vagal systems.

The polyvagal perspective of view is an endeavor to apply builds got from the Polyvagal Theory to understand the disparities in the writing identified with the technique for estimation, neurophysiological and neuroanatomical systems, and versatile elements of vagal efferent pathways. The methodology accentuates that predispositions or order fantasies happen when analysis are restricted to mental or physiological degrees of request. The polyvagal point of view recommends that it is fundamental, not exclusively, to understand the vagal efferent activities on the heart from a neurophysiological degree of request. Yet, the versatile capacity of the neural guidelines of the heart must be deciphered inside the setting of the phylogeny of the autonomic nervous system.

UNDERSTANDING THE YOGA THERAPY AND POLYVAGAL THEORY

Yoga therapy is a recently rising, self-managing complementary, and integrative healthcare (CIH) practice. It is developing in its professionalization, acknowledgment, and usage with a showed duty to setting practice standards, instructive and accreditation standards, and elevating analysis to help its viability for different populaces and conditions. Be that as it may, heterogeneity of training, poor detailing standards, and absence of a comprehensively acknowledged understanding of the neurophysiological components engaged with yoga therapy confines the organizing of testable speculations and clinical applications. Currently proposed structures of yoga-put together practices center concerning the coordination of base up neurophysiological and top-down neurocognitive instruments. Moreover, it has been suggested that phenomenology and first individual moral request can give a focal point through which yoga therapy is seen as a procedure that contributes towards eudaimonia prosperity in the experience of torment, disease, or incapacity. In this book, we expand on these systems and propose a model of yoga therapy that combines with Polyvagal Theory (PVT). PVT joins the development of the autonomic nervous system to the rise of prosocial practices and sets that the neural stages supporting social conduct are associated with looking after wellbeing, development, and rebuilding. This illustrative model, which interfaces neurophysiological examples of autonomic guidelines and articulation of enthusiastic and social conduct, is progressively used as a system for understanding human conduct, stress, and ailment. In particular, we portray how PVT can be conceptualized as a neurophysiological partner to the yogic ideal of the gunas, or characteristics of nature. Like the neural stages characterized in PVT, the gunas give the establishment from which conduct, passionate, and physical qualities develop. We depict how these two diverse yet practically equivalent to systems—one situated in neurophysiology and the other in an old-fashioned knowledge convention—feature yoga therapy's advancement of physical, mental, and social prosperity for self-guideline and versatility. This parallel between the neural foundation of PVT and the gunas of yoga is instrumental in making a translational structure for yoga therapy to line up with its philosophical establishments. Thusly, yoga therapy can work as an unmistakable practice as opposed to fitting into an outside model for its usage in examine and clinical settings.

Yoga therapy is proposed to encourage eudaimonic prosperity with its numerous impacts for physical, mental, and social wellbeing for assorted populaces through the structure of self-administrative abilities and developing versatility of the system. The qualities of the gunas of yoga and the neural foundation of the PVT, while not the equivalent, are reflected in each other.

Accordingly, working with gunas and neural stages that underlie physical, mental, and social characteristics give a procedure to the use of yoga rehearses for encouraging systemic guidelines and strength.

Yoga therapy manufactures a solid establishment in sattva and the neural foundation of the VVC for the rise of connection, peacefulness, and eudaimonia with coming about advantages to physiological, mental, and conduct wellbeing and prosperity. What's more, strength is encouraged through changing the relationship to the common vacillations of the gunas of rajas and tamas, and their neural partner foundation of SNS and DVC, with the end goal that the individual figures out how to successfully "bob back" to conditions of rebuilding and assemble versatility.

It is when yoga is rehearsed and comprehended as a firm and far-reaching system that the advantages for self-guideline and versatility might be figured it out. As one adapts new reactions to potential BME stressors, the individual may encounter more noteworthy physiological, mental, and conduct wellbeing and prosperity. The assembly of PVT and the gunas may help outline yoga therapy as a strategy that supports self-guideline, strength, and for diminishing allostatic load through building solid relationships to BME marvels. At the point when yoga therapy is applied through this viewpoint of moving fundamental guna states and neural stages, the incorporated idea of the training can be comprehended as particular from other CIH rehearses. It is trusted that this helps advise both research and healthcare settings keen on coordinating yoga mediations for different patient populaces and conditions.

THE IMPORTANCE OF POLYVAGAL THEORY

For specialists, and pop-brain research devotee the same, understanding polyvagal theory can help with:

- Getting trauma and PTSD

- Understanding the movement of assault and withdrawal in relationships

- Seeing how extraordinary pressure prompts separation or shutting down

- Seeing how to peruse body language

We like to think about our feelings as ethereal, complicated, and hard to order and recognize. In all actuality, feelings are reactions to a stimulus (inside or outside). Regularly they occur out of our mindfulness, particularly on the off chance that we are distant, or incongruent, with our inward enthusiastic life. Our base wants to remain alive is more essential to our body than even our capacity to consider staying alive. That is the place polyvagal theory comes in to play.

The nervous system is continually running out of sight, controlling our body capacities so we can consider different things—like what sort of frozen yoghurt we'd prefer to request, or how to get that A in medical school. The whole nervous system works pair with the brain and can assume control over our passionate experience, regardless of whether we don't need it to.

Animals are an incredible case of how we handle pressure, since they respond basely, without mindfulness. They do what we would if we weren't so very much restrained. If you've ever watched a National Geographic Africa extraordinary, you've seen a lioness pursue a gazelle. A gathering of gazelles is brushing, and abruptly one gazes upward, hyper-mindful of what's going on around him: the entire group get notified and focuses. After a minute, the lioness begins her pursuit. The gazelle she's singled out runs as quickly as possible (sympathetic nervous system) until he is gotten. At the point when he is reached, he in a flash goes limp (parasympathetic nervous system).

The lioness hauls the gazelle back to her fledglings, where they start to play with it before they go in for the murder. If that the lioness gets distracted, and the gazelle sees an opportunity, he's up. He runs off once more, appearing as though he all of a sudden returned to life (again into sympathetic nervous system reaction). At the point when the gazelle was gotten, with teeth around his neck, his shutdown reaction kicked in—he solidified. At the point when he saw the chance to run, his battle or flight kicked in, and he ran. The polyvagal theory covers those three states—connection, fight or flight, or shutdown.

The connection mode

During non-unpleasant circumstances, if we are genuinely sound, our bodies remain in a social engagement state, or a cheerful, ordinary, non-go ballistic state.

I like to call it a "connection." By connection, I imply that we are equipped for "connected" cooperation with another individual. We are strolling near, unafraid, making the most of our day, eating with loved ones and our body and feelings feel typical. It's additionally called ventral vagal reaction since that is the piece of the brain that is initiated during connection mode. It resembles a green light for an ordinary life.

<u>What does this look like and feel?</u>

- Our safe system is sound.

- We feel ordinary bliss, transparency, harmony, and interest in existence.

- We are resting soundly and eating typically.

- Our face is expressive.

- We genuinely identify with others.

- We all the more effectively comprehend and tune in to other people.

- Our body feels quiet and grounded.

<u>The fight or flight mode</u>

The sympathetic nervous system is our prompt response to stretch that influences each organ in the body. The sympathetic nervous system causes that "fight or flight" state we have all known about. It gives us those prompts so it can keep us alive.

How does this occur? What does this look like and feel?

- We sense to risk and stick to check the surroundings for genuine threat.

- We discharge cortisol, epinephrine and norepinephrine to help us achieve what we have to—escape, or fight our foe.

- Our heartbeat spikes, we sweat, and we feel more assembled.

- We feel restless, apprehensive, or irate.

- There might be flashes of outward appearances of dread and outrage, with the foundation of all the more a still face. On the off chance that positive feelings are available, they typically look constrained.

- Our assimilation backs off as blood hurries to the muscles.

- Our blood vessels choke to the digestive organs and widen to the muscles expected to run or fight.

- We might need to flee, or punch somebody, or respond physically here and there, or simply puff-up and look unnerving.

- Our muscles may feel tense, electric, tight, vibrating, throbbing, trembling, and hard.

- Our hands might be moist.

- Our stomach might be agonizingly hitched.

- All our faculties center.

- Our motions may show guarding of our imperative organs, clench hands held, or puffing ourselves up to look more significant or more grounded.

In fight or flight, at some level, we accept we can, in any case, endure whatever risk we believe is perilous.

The shutdown mode

What's fascinating about this piece of the parasympathetic nervous system? It can keep us solidified as a versatile component to help us get by to either fight or flight once more. At the point when a lion assaulted David Livingston, he later revealed, "it caused a kind of vagueness in which there was no feeling of torment nor sentiment of dread, however very aware of every one of that was going on."

At the point when our sympathetic nervous system has kicked into overdrive, despite everything we can't escape and feel approaching passing the dorsal vagal parasympathetic nervous system takes control. It causes freezing or shutdown, as to a type of self-conservation. (Consider somebody who drops under extreme pressure.)

<u>What does this look like and feel?</u>

- Emotionally, it feels like separation, deadness, bleary-eyed, sadness, disgrace, a feeling of feeling caught, out of the body, disengaged from the world.

- Our eyes may watch fixed and scattered.

- The dorsal engine core through the unmyelinated vagus nerve diminishes our pulse, blood pressure, outward appearances, sexual and invulnerable reaction systems.

- We might be activated to feel disgusted, hurl, poop, immediately pee.

- We may feel low or no agony.

- Our lungs (bronchi) choke, and we inhale more slow.

- We may experience issues getting words out or feel narrowing around our throat.

- Our brain has diminished digestion, and this causes lost body mindfulness, limp appendages, diminished capacity to think unmistakably, and diminished the ability to set down story recollections.

- Our body stance may fall or twist up in a ball.

In shutdown mode, at some level, our nervous system accepts we are in a dangerous circumstance, and it attempts to keep us alive through keeping our body still. A few people who have had both connection trauma and ensuing trauma can have interminable suicidality and separation scenes that last days to months. Research shows that extended haul arrangements include:

- Dialectical conduct treatment

- Mentalization-based treatment

- Transference centered treatment

CHAPTER TWO

DORSAL VAGAL, FREEZE, AND DISSOCIATIVE PAIN AND EFFECTIVE POLYVAGAL SOLUTIONS

The essential job of the dorsal vagal system, in people, is to direct organs underneath the stomach. In any case, that is by all account, not the only job. We should place it in context. Hereditarily, the dorsal vagal pathway of the autonomic nervous system is essentially fundamentally the same as what's been seen in hard fish and even cartilaginous fish. When it advanced to warm-blooded creatures, its job was indeed consigned principally to underneath the stomach.

This implies it controls fundamentally every one of those instinctive organs that we are truly not mindful of. Nonetheless, there are a few tracks, or pathways, that are still, one might say minimal, old systems that go to the heart and regions like the throat. If you somehow managed to animate the uttermost, most profound piece of your throat, that would be directed by the dorsal vagus. What occurs if you invigorate that piece of the throat? You disgorge. Spewing forth is, as it were is a dorsal vagal reaction. The system is genuinely going down, and this is an exceptionally versatile methodology for disposing of poisons and different things that might be happening. In the first place, when we talk about the dorsal vagal system, it starts in the brain stem region called the dorsal engine core of the vagus or all the more regularly now known as the dorsal core of the vagus. A portion of the pathways move through the core vague and then return through the vagus and a part of those that relocated wind up being a piece of the core uncertain or the ventral vagus, when you see it originating from the brain stem, you mostly have a brought together coordinated nerve.

Many individuals feel that they're two separate nerves, the ventral vagus and the dorsal vagus; in any case, they're actually across the board conductor, and we need to imagine that. There are just about 15% of the filaments in that channel. 15% to 20% of those strands are efferent filaments significance going down from the brain. Of that 15%, 80% of those are setting off to the dorsal vagus, and not many are heading off to the ventral vagus. So extremely, the transcendent highlights of our vagal system are managing sub-diaphragmatic organs. The significant part that we genuinely need to get to when we start examining torment is this job of the afferents, of these systems, being the tactile part returning to the brain.

So the dorsal vagus originates from a zone that is dorsal to the core questionable, which is ventral to the dorsal.

We utilize the polyvagal system as a sort of neural guide to investigate torment differently than it is typically talked about. The polyvagal theory is a conspicuous method for sorting out data. Be that as it may, with that method for arranging data, it makes a translating strategy to understand the human experience and to help start treating agony and trauma.

THE ROLE OF THE DORSAL VAGAL AND PAIN

Holding those particular subtleties is truly not significant because they're incredibly unimportant to understanding the capacity. The capacity that we start understanding is that the core ambiguous vagal filaments are connected with the face and influence that we typically have, while the dorsal vagal strands are all the more transcendently connected to regions beneath the stomach. Gastric agony, bad-tempered entrail, every one of these things that are truly side effects of different disorders that numerous individuals who endure trauma have, are truly markers of a typical guideline of the dorsal vagus. This turns out to be extraordinarily significant because, inside the model of the Polyvagal Theory, both the sympathetic nervous system and the dorsal vagus can be enrolled as resistance systems. At the point when the ventral vagus is truly working at a significant level and controlling great, at that point, the sympathetic is the only piece of the homeostatic procedures. They bolster wellbeing, development, and reclamation. They likewise bolster development without being a protection system.

THE DORSAL VAGAS AND NOCICEPTION AS A CAUSE OF PAIN

Stephen clarifies there's a ton of implanted research skimming around in neurophysiology on the relationship between the afferents of the dorsal vagus and nociception (the encoding and handling of hurtful improvements in the nervous system, and in this way the body's capacity to detect potential mischief). Something revealed in writing is that the substantial piece of the vagus cooperates with a spinal pathway that is engaged with nociception. That gets fascinating as far as builds or ideas like fibromyalgia, which will, in general, be connected especially with individuals who have encountered profound shutdown and are truly coasting between a dorsal state and a sympathetic state. They're shutting down. If you just followed their colon you'd likely observe a similar marvel. One might say going among clogging and looseness of the bowels; you'd locate the same similitude at a lower level. What you need to understand is that several things get indeed activated because of the changing in the afferent guideline of the autonomic nervous system while in a dorsal vagal state. That implies that the system that manages blood pressure guideline, the baroreceptors, gets disturbed. Individuals often get unsteady and drop.

They become "vasovagal sympathetic," they fall, and this is because of vagal afferents. It's a system that isn't connected, so just a piece of it is working. Individuals displaying these issues often may have posterial hypotension or hypertension. It's the blood pressure guideline. Hess found the connection between eternal weariness disorder and blood pressure guideline issues that they are a piece of a similar system.

We may have three disorders connected regarding symptomatology. One is constant weariness which will be an indication of numerous individuals who have trauma or who have encountered drawn-out periods in dorsal vagal states. The second is blood pressure guideline, not hypertension, yet truly getting discombobulated when standing up. This isn't the sort of discombobulation where things are turning, however where the individual truly begins hitting the ground. The third connection is fibromyalgia. These are no different system - fibromyalgia, incessant weakness, and blood pressure guideline - that has gone hypotensive. This is all piece of the dorsal vagus system, in a sense, being the final retreat and being utilized in a guarded mode.

These 3 challenges are features of a similar disorder. A specialist from the U.K. sent

Stephen a letter concerning a customer whom he said: "seems to have a polyvagal disorder." Stephen chose to deconstruct these manifestations so we can discuss every one of these side effects and how they would depict fibromyalgia, blood pressure guideline, and ceaseless exhaustion. On the off chance that the individual is spending a lot of their neuro-guideline time in a dorsal vagal express that isn't secured with the highlights of safety, we can't immobilize unafraid.

<u>FEAR AND DEPRESSION, POLYVAGAL SCIENCE, AND PAIN</u>

Subside needs to underscore dread and depression as far as polyvagal science and torment. All the time when the agony gets constant, the adjustment to allostatic load (the mileage on the body because of incessant stress) is to move towards a shutdown. This happens because there is dread related to the heap and depression that will, in general, fortify itself. Regularly in creatures that are undermined, or under life, danger won't move. They give off an impression of being dead — much the same as a gazelle that will be brought down by a cheetah. There's no development yet then minutes after the fact the creature jumps up and goes off on its way. Since those states are typically time-restricted. However, when you bring dread into the immobility circuit, it keeps up immobility or freeze, yet keeps up it vigorously.

How about we take a guinea pig for a model. At the point when you take the guinea pig and grasp it, it gets stable. At that point in almost no time, seconds to minutes, it springs up and goes off. Be that as it may, on the off chance that you startle it each time it goes in, it remains longer. What could be five minutes or seven seconds, with the dread included, can keep it uncertainly. Diminish analyzed that in Brazil and had the creature remain in that state for 24 hours. Some of the time, creatures will pass on.

DANGERS AND BENEFITS IN COMING OUT OF IMMOBILITY

At the point when an individual start to leave immobility, clinically, there's a surge of hyper excitement. Stephen was discussing the sympathetic and dorsal vagal system being in this sort of flip-flop. What you need to do is help the individual contain the sympathetic system, by keeping them connected socially in the present time and place. At that point, there is a guideline, and the stable individual can leave the immobility, out of the dorsal vagal shut down, because they're not reactivating themselves. If the agony turns out to be increasingly intense, you need to state "OK.

On the off chance that that agony turns out to be progressively intense and you start to see that somewhat more, you notice if it's proceeding to increment if it's beginning to diminish or on the off chance that it continues as before or if it changes to something different". With this sort of greeting, customers get the feeling that time moves along and blast, before they know it, they've left from the immobility state.

Stephen proceeds to clarify that a few warm-blooded creatures, through phylogenetic advancement, can go all through polyvagal responses as versatile capacities. Little rodents likewise do this: be that as it may, even in going into the dorsal vagal reaction for a bit of rat, there's a danger of dropping dead. The equivalent is valid with the guinea pig; there is an opportunity merely dropping dead from the immobilization reaction. This probability will, in general, happen with mice and other little rodents. What seems, by all accounts, to be versatile can likewise be deadly; as warm-blooded animals, we need heaps of oxygen, and when we go into shutdown states, we're not supporting our life needs just as our body needs.

Another part to recollect is the thought of when the creatures leave dorsal vagal states, they shut down, and they get profoundly immobilized. There is additionally a feeling of a thoroughly prepared state for some versatile reasons, and one is to get away. They are attempting to recover the blood into their muscles, once again into their bodies, so they currently have the suitable metabolic assets to move the muscles. You have these jerks and different things that are occur4ing as you refuel the body. At that point, the guideline begins happening. For whatever length of time that people who have recently experienced closed down are prepared, which implies that they are in a condition of frenzy or mayhem, they won't shut down. You need to consider these to be as having versatile highlights. They are not so many highlights of good social association, yet they keep them out of shutting down. Our nervous system has advanced, flawlessly and smoothly to move among assembly and social communication. That characterizes how vertebrates work and advance and endure because they needed to recognize quickly, who was sheltered and who was undependable.

THE DORSAL VAGUS, GOODNESS, AND HELP WITH PAIN

Diminish follows up a prior dialogue to speak all the more explicitly about the way that numerous therapists, when they find out about the dorsal vagal system, and its focal job in trauma and incessant torment, will consider it to be the adversary. It's practically similar to "well if we could remove it, is there any valid reason why you wouldn't simply remove it?" Why not cut out those afferent and efferent connections? The explanation is that the dorsal vagal system in well-evolved creatures or people is exceptionally fundamental to essential sentiments of goodness and additionally bolsters sentiments of connection through the ventral vagal system. At the point when you feel warm and upbeat, you can get an aching "God; it'd be magnificent on the off chance that we could return to our strolls on the sea shore and so forward." Feelings of happiness and those emotions, they originate from the gut. They originate from the stomach, and they originate from the heart. What we're discussing is a system that is so essential for our very own working, yet can so promptly get maladaptive and therapists need to understand and hold together the two sides of this.

Correspondingly, Stephen has had therapists ask "Wouldn't we be able to remove it? Wouldn't we be able to discourage it?" He accepts that they are feeling the loss of the entire understanding of what's happening and that is the reason if that system is utilized as a guarded system, it can't be a system that supports our homeostatic needs.

The equivalent is valid for the sympathetic. To conceptualize this present, a term wasn't preferred much called "Autonomic Balance." Autonomic Balance alluded to the way that it might be said you have sympathetic enough, and enough parasympathetic. Instead, Stephen accentuates that "On the off chance that the ventral vagal circuit is truly working great, at that point sub diaphragmatically you have [organically] autonomic harmony between the sympathetic and the dorsal vagus." This is the sort of equalization you need to have, and this advances positive sentiments. He notes what Peter was underscoring was an inclination of prosperity and how that climbs the afferent vagus from the gut and indeed commands our capacity to get to various zones of our brain. We should not overlook this monstrous progression of tangible data that is principally originating from underneath the stomach that is changing the availability to different pieces of our brain. It's a screen.

<u>HANDY WAYS OF SHIFTING OUT OF THE FREEZE</u>

Peter has discovered that occasionally it's conceivable to do various things with preparing. He has a gadget that resembles a little trampoline, yet it's unique. It doesn't utilize any springs, and it has flexible bungee strings. Presently when somebody stands on this, one arrives at a spot where he/she starts to, as it were, have a collaboration with the trampoline. It feels like, among you, that the trampoline needs to move you a tad, to bob you a little minuscule piece, and because you think that ricocheting, you're getting new proprioceptive data, activating data from the joints, from the muscles.

Peter works with individuals in extreme shut down, and accepts that doing verbal therapy could go on until the following century! Only getting these little developments on this trampoline takes them out enough, so they're available to versatility, and you can work with them. It's great to recollect that there are non-verbal and development arranged methods for doing this. Stephens' point of view is consistently to deconstruct what is by all accounts attempting to give it a physiological approval.

Where instincts appear to be genuinely on target, would we be able to give a motivation behind why? There are two things. One is shaking. A lot of people who have these encounters will frequently do something like this, and they need to understand that they are invigorating vagal afferents and attempting to manage blood pressure through the development of their bodies in space. It's not merely body and space. They are animating the carotid baroreceptors. It's calming for individuals to shake. We need to consider it to be a neural exercise, as an endeavor to restore a system that has been down managed.

Another way brings up the entire issue of the pelvic floor. A ton of people who have trauma encounters understand that vast numbers of these trauma encounters will be precisely related, particularly stomach medical procedure or sub-stomach medical procedure. The pelvic floor is going to; it could be said, quit working. We need to understand that the pelvic floor is, as a representation, a stomach. Similarly, as our stomach is to our lungs, the pelvic floor is to our bladder and colon. It makes a negative weight. The pelvic floor contracts, so everybody who has had pelvic floor issues is told, "Do Kegel exercises." But Kegel exercises are sphincter muscles. The pelvic floor isn't a sphincter muscle; it has sphincter muscles navigating it. The issue is, how you would get the pelvic floor to change and work? You do that through moving equalization or parity challengers. This resembles the methodology with the trampoline. We may likewise utilize the BOSU, which is half of an exercise ball.

Peter concurs that merely sitting on a gymnastic ball and making little developments, and then finding support to discover the sentiment of giving up the pelvic floor into the ball can truly move things. On the off chance that the individual enables the ball to help the pelvic stomach, at that point, the stomach unwinds into the ball. You see this frequently with sexual trauma, stomach medical procedures, and so forward.

Stephen saw that Peter shut his eyes while depicting this procedure. His eyes began to hang and close. That helped Stephen to remember the way that he had a medical procedure and I didn't care for what they guided him to do, to manage the pelvic floor issues, so he made his very own model. He additionally understood that on the off chance that he shut his eyes, it was increasingly troublesome and testing, and it was working better since he was not utilizing the viewable prompts. It's ideal for working with customers with their eyes open and something to clutch. It makes a connectedness if you are with someone else. You can even give them your arm to clutch with the goal that when they leave shut down, there you are.

PHYSICAL RESOURCES OF THE DORSAL VAGAL

From Stephen's point of view, it's a troublesome inquiry. As it were, it's our center or our base of being alive, and the issue is that when we attempt to utilize it as an asset, it's practically similar to using it as a safeguard. Instead, we need to; it could be said to support it. At the point when we sustain it, it serves us, and this is the place the afferents are returning, saying, "all reasonable." The "every reasonable" afferent are similar afferents that help our capacity to connect with others and our ability to get to different zones of the brain that are both social and innovative. On the off chance that the sign from the dorsal vagus is, "I'm in a tough situation," it will down manage everything else. It's an emotionally supportive network, an asset system, whereby giving, we get, rather than a feeling of abuse from it.

Maggie proposes returning to Peter's recommendation of standing on one portion of an exercise ball and having something to clutch and having somebody there. Doesn't getting security make a vast difference? Stephen concurs wellbeing and trust change into a neural exercise of development instead of a shutting down protective response.

CHAPTER THREE

SIGNIFICANCE OF VENTRAL VAGAL ACTIVITY TO FORESTALL DEFENSE AND SHUTDOWN

Essentially a similar representation works for the dorsal vagus. The dorsal vagus is fundamental; it is anything but an awful system; however, it's not beneficial for that system to be utilized or enrolled as a guard. That turns out to be extremely, the essential issue and the Polyvagal Theory gives you the hierarchical model. It says, as long as the ventral vagus is truly in command or running, at that point your sympathetic can move any way they need in a progressively homeostatic manner to advance bloodstream and advance solid development and reclamation. It's just when the ventral vagus gets withdrawn that we at that point get into this weakness of a sympathetic resistance system. At the point when that doesn't work, well, at that point the dorsal vagus is the main thing you have left, and that closes you down. You start seeing the hierarchical way that things work.

What is hugely significant is the job of the vagal afferents from the gut, from the sub stomach. Their job in the balance of torment is a piece of this current section's accentuation. Peter noticed the way that the vagus nerve, the biggest nerve in the entire human body is 80% afferent, when we see what happens when individuals stall out in the dorsal vagal system. Steve has stressed its administrative capacity, both the dorsal vagal and the sympathetic, and the ventral vagal. In any case, there are numerous circumstances, especially trauma and torment - where this guideline isn't generally homeostatic, where it's maladaptive.

PROCEDURES TO SHIFT OUT OF MALADAPTIVE DEFENSE STATES

One of the manners in which that we can change out of those maladaptive states, because of trauma or agony, is through invigorating these afferents. There are a few different ways - one, for instance, is the utilization, of vibrating a sound, directly from the instinctive territory where you appear to be animating those afferents. Now and then you'll see an individual go from shut down and into balance. Sympathetic hyper excitement is a vital part of this substantial autonomic example of supporting, of choking, of holding. This prompts torment, and that torment itself brings on additional supporting and further enactment of the sympathetic system. At the point when the propping design and the pain itself have become increasingly intense, the body closes down additional into what Steve

has discussed as a metabolic retreat, a

condition of vitality protection.

Simultaneously, that upgrades the arrival of

endorphins, which are the body's own

narcotic agony mitigating system.

<u>MOVING OUT OF SHUTDOWN AND WORKING WITH THE SYMPATHETIC RESPONSES</u>

Underneath it could be said, individual

movements from intense torment, to intense,

moving towards constant, and that is the

sympathetic excitement/supporting example.

At that point, after some time, it goes into

the shutdown. To help individuals, when

they've been in the shutdown, we need to figure out how to help get them a tad out of the shutdown and then utilize the sympathetic response under that. As Steve was stating, a ton of that guideline originates from that ventral vagal social engagement system, by the therapist truly being available and having the option to direct them through those excitement sensations.

Stephen and Peter concur on the significant mediation of paunch breathing or stomach relaxing. A large number of the incredibly ground-breaking afferents identified with relaxing for the ventral vagal system are inserted in the stomach. The issue is, we can utilize an intentional system, which means control of the stomach and breathing, or if nothing else deliberate breathing, to drive the stomach down and to broaden the span of exhalations just as to improve or expand stomach relaxing. That, as it were, expands the ventral vagal stream. Once more, the essential basic topic here is that the sympathetic in the dorsal vagal system will work in an impressive homeostatic manner as long as the ventral vagus is genuinely working. Subside has appeared in an excellent way that you can recover a portion of this control through a willful breathing technique

Since what that is doing is practically setting off the ventral vagus to empower the dorsal vagus and the sympathetic to return into a homeostatic circumstance. Propping, which, is an increment in engine tone, is a sympathetic preparation and that has transient impacts. As Peter recommends, "In case I'm gripping my clench hands and planning, I am essentially saying to my ventral vagal system, 'Leave since I'm in a barrier mode.' Now, if this doesn't dispose of the torment, since I'm in a hierarchical system, or I am a hierarchical system, I've just discarded, disposed of the ventral vagus as an alternative. On the off chance that this doesn't work, what does my nervous system do? It goes down to its most reduced level."

We can't state that all the dorsal vagal reactions are adverse because there is a level of absence of pain, and once in a while, there is separation and no sentiment of agony. Be that as it may, the expense to the social association is a cataclysmic cost to pay. As Peter notes, when working with a customer, it's essential to respect and regard the requirement for that specific barrier system and then continuously help the customer to move out of it to a less, more hierarchically contemporary system, a present time and place system. Maggie brings up that a lot of therapists downgrade the freeze reaction and are practically phobic about it. They don't need the customer to be in a frozen state. It's imperative to realize what sort of psycho-instruction we can give customers about how the freeze has been vital to them.

Peter includes that the freeze is a versatile reaction, implying that it has the versatile capacity and that is a piece of the psycho instructive part. At the point when individuals begin to understand that their body has responded, truly, in a predictable and versatile way, it's not deliberate conduct. You can say "Well, master, I on the off chance that I would not like to close down, I shouldn't have closed down." But shut down is anything but a willful system. The body is getting things done outside the domains of mindfulness. Although we don't know about the triggers that put us into these physiological states, the afferent input of our physiological moves surely are inside the domain of our mindfulness.

The issue is, how we would name those physiological reactions? Do we disclose to ourselves that we accomplished something incorrectly or do we attempt to state, "Look, my body's accomplishing something? It might have been successful for an intense, versatile reaction, however clearly in the ceaseless one, the body should be re-taught to state 'Hello, it's protected, leave there.' Another significant factor is that when somebody leaves the shutdown, you usually hear, "I didn't hurt that much previously." When the separation and the absence of pain break down, there's torment both physically and inwardly. As professionals, we need to utilize instruction that fundamentally clarifies it that way. At that point, we must be available and accessible to help them at that point work through the agony. Nothing is settled – agony and trauma issues don't resolve when the individual's in the shutdown- - that will possibly occur on the off chance that they need to turn out enough to enable them to be vigorously open.

Diminish concurs that therapists are often awkward with the shutdown to organize. This is likely because of a couple of elements. One is if therapists are terrified of the freeze in themselves, of their inside state. Another is that they don't have a clue what to do. Most therapists are caring; they're giving it a second thought and by and large well-tuned in for the customers. If that is everything they do, in any case, it won't be adequate for somebody who's in a shutdown state

CHAPTER FOUR

DEVELOPMENT OF POLYVAGAL THEORY: HIERARCHICAL PATTERNS

The polyvagal theory is an understanding of the summarization of our developmental history. For warm-blooded creatures, the transformative history is called phylogeny, which thinks about the nervous systems (or their highlights) that we've acquired from our progenitors. For this situation, the progenitors are reptiles, land and water proficient, and fish. As vertebrates, we have acquired a ton of circuits. As these circuits change, they brought about practical neuro-stages for huge numbers of the practices we as people express. One thing we have overlooked or didn't understand until the polyvagal theory empowered us to have the reconceptualization, was our remarkable progress from reptiles to warm-blooded creatures. In that progress from antiquated reptiles to even the crude vertebrates, there are sure things that happened.

Those things are tied in with empowering co-guideline one might say, empowering one well-evolved creature to help manage the physiological condition of another vertebrate. That required prompting, or the social engagement, of another with sign of wellbeing and the, with those signs of security, to empower two of the species to be agreeable in one another's quality. The entire history of warm-blooded animals is tied in with being agreeable within sight of another or another fitting well-evolved creature. It's truly what gets disturbed with trauma. At the point when trauma happens, individuals are never again ready to co-direct with another, since often the trauma has been incurred by another person, and their nervous system currently doesn't welcome the other individual into their essence. The polyvagal model truly has three polyvagal states, including the crudest system that we've acquired, which is imparted to for all intents and purposes all vertebrates. It returns to the ligament that fish have, that is identified with the capacity to immobilize with dread, and to utilize fixed status as a protection system.

This gets one of the basic focuses – that is, people who have gone into a breakdown or a demise faking, have changed because they've gained access to this extremely, antiquated circuit. Hereditarily, the following stage that advanced was the activation system, which we as a whole know as fight-flight. Be that as it may, fight-flight additionally has certain awesome focal points, because as long as we continue moving, we're not going to be powerless against closed down or breakdown. You see those side effects of numerous individuals who have trauma chronicles. Being in a physiological condition of fight-flight isn't awesome for one's body. It prompts ailments. It's likewise shocking for social associations since we need to signal others to, one might say, remain quiet, co-control, and offer encounters.

We could utilize the term between emotional encounters. We need to share considerations and thoughts and be available with another. With the coming of warm-blooded animals, a more current circuit went ahead, and this is what we're marking either the ventral vagal circuit or the social engagement system. The social engagement system was connecting the neuro-guideline of the considerable number of muscles, the strident muscles that control the face and head – including the muscles of vocalization, the muscles of tuning in, the muscles of prompting in the face, and the muscles of how we articulate the prosodic highlights in our voice with the vagal guideline of the heart. We essentially are continually wearing our face on our heart, and we're passing on our physiological state in our voice. We recognize the physiological condition of others, through their voices and with their appearances. When we watch somebody, we get signals on the speaker's face, tuning in to their voice and choosing, is this an agreeable individual to hear? Or then again would it be advisable for me to consider the words, or would it be a good idea for me to consider the emotions that the words pass on? So the social engagement system is truly what makes people human, or makes warm-blooded animal's well-evolved creature. Your canine has a truly all around created social engagement system and numerous felines do too; they pass on their sentiments in their vocalizations, in their outward appearances, in their signals, and even how they move their heads.

The social engagement system is this awesome capacity to pass on to another what our physiological state is. What the polyvagal theory assembles is the view that these circuits are hierarchical. Hierarchical implies that more current circuits can hinder the more established ones. This means social engagement can down-manage fight-flight and can quiet us down similarly as fight-flight can keep us out of shutting down. There are three levels, and every one restrains the cruder system underneath it. The word that was utilized to portray this is a word called "disintegration," which originates from researcher John Hughlings Jackson, who was exceptionally intrigued by brain forms and in this restraint of brain circuits, with the goal that they become progressively crude and receptive when we have brain harm or ailment. So, the autonomic nervous system works a similar way. Our most up to date circuit quiets us; our more seasoned circuits can be utilized for a guard. What enables social engagement to happen while the guarded systems of fight-flight are being handicapped? Stephen utilizes the expression "highlight finders" that fundamentally accept that our nervous system developed to recognize includes in the other, to help us distinguish wellbeing and to quiet us down. So those component identifiers are a piece of the build he calls "neuroception." You can't discuss the social engagement system without discussing neuroception. Perception is the instrument through which our nervous system identifies wellbeing and then empowers the social engagement system to work. It recognizes this without mindfulness. It is a different system since it isn't the personal mindfulness we are in a safe environment.

Our nervous system is identifying the degree of security; at that point, the physiology reacts. One can be extremely mindful of their physiology. Much like setting off to talk, we go in, and we state "Well, the words sound great or if nothing else if I somehow managed to understand it, it would be great, yet you know, there is something in particular about that individual that I don't generally feel good with." Everyone has had those issues. It is difficult to name; however, we feel awkward, perhaps it's an absence of prosody in that individual's voice, the absence of engagement. We could state it is the absence of being extremely touchy or having the feeling that the other is being a legitimate individual. It's actually that the words are there, yet the emotions underneath the words may not be. That is the thing that our bodies are reacting to. We react all the more profoundly to weakening of voice than we do to what is said by the individual. At the point when our body reacts, we feel it and then build up our very own account. That is how we either feel that we can be near individuals, or we feel that we ought to be truly separating. The hidden subject here is, there is no social engagement, except if our neuroception gets the highlights of wellbeing.

HOW THE NERVOUS SYSTEM DETECTS SAFETY:

Specifically, how does the nervous system identify these components of safety? It's unmistakably more explicit than we give our nervous system acknowledgement for. We believe it's a complicated procedure - you have to go to class to learn it, you have to look about miniaturized scale includes in the internal pieces of the eyes, or you have to do outline by-outline investigation. Be that as it may, by and large, our body's getting profound things like the sound of voice. The best model utilized is Bill Clinton. Clinton's voice was amazingly prosodic. There used to be these accounts circumventing Capitol Hill that, not about the ladies, additionally fascinating is the narratives that returned from the Republicans who had gone to the White House. They would make some great memories, they would connect with Bill Clinton, and they would leave not realizing what they had consented to. They were getting these prompts, and they had thoroughly down controlled their barriers. This turns into a genuine intriguing thing. The other alternative is George W. Shrub. He didn't balance the recurrence of the inflection. He tweaked uproar. Along these lines, he seemed, by all accounts, to be yapping at you and conversing with accentuation. This had the impact of pushing individuals away. For those two, it had little to do with the substance. As educated people, we state it had an inseparable tie to the substance; however, it had a great deal to do with how they had the option to impart.

Our nervous system is identifying the prosodic highlights (the arrangement of discourse factors including musicality, speed, pitch, and relative accentuation that recognizes vocal patterns), and this is amazing. Although we can close our eyes when we would prefer not to take a gander at something, we experience issues shutting our ears. This entry is so incredible, particularly for individuals with trauma accounts. They experience problems looking taking a gander at somebody; however, they can't kill their nervous system's capacity to decipher prosodic highlights of voice. It's designed in. For an individual with a trauma history, a hand signal can be confused. On the off chance that you have a pooch, and a more interesting comes and puts a hand over the line of vision, the canine will react. We need to feel that people have a portion of these highlights. We need to perceive what's before us. We would prefer not to see things behind us. If we become at all awkward in the physical circumstance, we come hyper-careful about what's happening behind us, and we're stiff with the connection. Social engagement is subject to how we control the muscles of our countenances and heads. If we state that in case we're physically and physiologically preparing data as safety, our face turns out to be suddenly captivating, instead of a bogus grin, which underlines the lower some portion of the face. In any case, it's the upper piece of our face that is giving us the signals to safety.

The contemporary culture reminds us that individuals use Botox to hose their wrinkles; however, the wrinkles are a method for disclosing to us that individuals are genuinely intrigued by what we are stating. The Botox may dispose of the wrinkles, yet it likewise makes an issue. As an aside, if you manage guardians or kids or grown-ups who have a chemical imbalance, one of the remarks that we hear is "Well, my child he looks so youthful he doesn't have a wrinkle." What they are misunderstanding is that a considerable lot of the wrinkles are a sign of neuro guideline of the muscles there beneath the skin, particularly the orbital muscle called the orbicularis oculi. In this way, the main standard isn't just that we can organize our muscles. Yet, on the off chance that we're in this physiological state, at that point, the suddenness happens, and there's a significant distinction between unconstrained grins and constrained grins. Our nervous system recognizes this quickly, and that is a piece of why we don't feel good with specific sorts of individuals. Much the same as during political decision time, the bogus grins of people truly is a significant mood killer to our nervous system.

Stephen utilizes a slide in his discussions that shows an antiquated Chinese veil and one of the photos is an image of the cover of satisfaction. How you realize that its joy is that it has huge crow's feet as an afterthought. Thus, this was utilized as an unambiguous prompt to the crowd of satisfaction. The dermatologists are not educated in this data and individuals don't need their wrinkles. All things being equal, individuals put make-up on, particularly ladies, and I surmise men do a portion of this now as well, in an exceptionally static mode, they hold their face up. In any case, it's not the static method of the face that is alluring. It's the dynamic part of the face. That becomes mixed up in the way of life.

CHAPTER FIVE

UNDERSTANDING HOW TRAUMA AFFECT THE VAGUS NERVE

As people, we do a similar thing as that gazelle when we see passionate or physical risk. We switch back and forth between gentle touching (parasympathetic - connection mode), fight or flight (sympathetic system-fight and flight) or shutdown (parasympathetic-shut down mode). Our reaction is all in our impression of the occasion. Possibly somebody was playing a game when they hopped out to startle us; however, we blacked out.

Whatever the explanation, regardless of whether the episode was purposeful or not, our body moved into shutdown mode, we enrolled it as a trauma. Our body moved into shutdown mode. Or then again, perhaps the trauma occasion was truly, dangerous, and our nervous system reacted suitably to the improvements.

Regardless of what the reason was, our brain accepted what was going on was hazardous enough that it made our body go into flight, flight, or shutdown mode. On the off chance that somebody has experienced such a traumatic occasion, that their body tips into shutdown reaction, any occasion that helps the individual to remember that dangerous event can trigger them into disconnection or separation once more. Individuals can even live in a condition of disconnection or shut down for a considerable length of time or months one after another.

Veterans frequently experience this during uproarious, abrupt commotions, for example, firecrackers or tempests. A lady who was assaulted may rapidly switch into hypervigilant or separated reaction on the off chance that she feels somebody is following her. Somebody who was mishandled may be activated when significantly someone else begins hollering.

The issue happens when we haven't prepared the first trauma so that the first trauma is settled. That is the thing that PTSD (post-traumatic pressure issue) is—our body's eruption to a little reaction, and either stuck in fight and flight or close down. Individuals who experience trauma and the shutdown reaction, as a rule, feel disgrace around their failure to act when their body didn't move. They regularly wish they would have battled more during those minutes.

A Vietnam vet may feel they bombed their allies who died around them while they stood, solidified in dread. An assault injured individual may feel the person in question didn't fight off their attacker since they hardened. A casualty of misuse may feel they quit attempting to get away from their abuser, and that they are frail or fizzled. Quite a bit of "stress" preparing, which trains individuals to keep on staying in fight and flight mode, means to keep individuals out of separation during reality or demise circumstances. Lamentably, these practices aren't essential past first-class sports groups or exceptional powers. The perfect measure of worry, with great recuperation, can lead our nervous systems into more elevated levels of adjustment.

UNDERSTANDING POSTTRAUMATIC STRESS (PTSD)

Posttraumatic stress (PTSD) is a typical response to traumatic or stressful occasions. Studies show 3.5% of the United States (U.S.) populace will encounter PTSD at whatever year. Practically 37% of these cases can be named "serious." Somebody with PTSD may remember a traumatic encounter through recollections and dreams. They may stay away from tokens of the trauma to anticipate passionate distress. PTSD can likewise include memory issues and an uplifted reactivity to one's environment.

PTSD takes numerous structures. It might occur because of a catastrophic event or an individual disaster. It might emerge following an encounter or years after the fact. Individuals of any sexual orientation, ethnicity, and foundation can encounter it. Posttraumatic stress is a treatable condition. Individuals with PTSD may wish to contact a therapist. Therapy can help individuals process distressing feelings and recollections. Understanding one's side effects are regularly the initial step to diminishing them.

WHAT CAUSES PTSD?

PTSD can happen after a physically or psychologically stressful occasion. Circumstances that may achieve PTSD include:

- Transportation mishaps

- Military battle

- Abusive behavior at home

- Sexual maltreatment or ambush

Vicarious trauma, for example, learning of the demise of a friend or family member or encountering an assault as an observer. During a stunning or startling occasion, it is reasonable to encounter a "fight or flight" reaction. Expanded adrenaline and stress can be essential for endurance in crises. Forceful feelings like resentment and dread are additionally standard. However, a few people will keep reacting to trauma long after the threat has passed. Their mind's prompt response to the crisis turns into a default design. Psychological well-being experts search for practices that have an enduring and unfavourable effect. At the point when somebody's reaction to trauma meddles with their day by day life, a conclusion of PTSD might be fitting.

<u>SYMPTOM OF PTSD</u>

The Diagnostic and Statistical Manual (DSM) diagrams four classes of PTSD side effects: re-encountering, evasion, excitement/reactivity, and comprehension/mind-set. To meet all requirements for a PTSD finding, an individual ought to have manifestations from every classification. Every one of the expressions more likely than not is available for at any rate one month.

1. Re-encountering manifestations (need in any event one):

- Recurring and meddlesome recollections of the trauma

- Flashbacks where the individual feels or goes about as though the trauma is repeating

- Disturbing or terrifying contemplations when looked with tokens of trauma.

- Nightmares

- Intense physiological responses to tokens of the trauma, for example, fast heartbeat and perspiring.

2. Evasion indications (need in any event one):

- Avoiding tokens of the traumatic experience, including individuals, circumstances, places, or items

- Repressing or disregarding feelings or considerations identified with the occasion

3. Excitement and reactivity side effects (need in any event two):

- Outbursts of outrage with little incitement

- Reckless or self-damaging conduct

- Startling effectively

- Anxiety or sentiment of being "anxious."

- Insomnia

- Difficulty concentrating

4. Comprehension or state of mind manifestations (need at any rate two):

- Inability to recollect a significant detail of the occasion

- Exaggerated negative convictions, for example, "I am terrible" or "nobody can be trusted."

- Feeling steady negative feelings like disgrace or frightfulness.

- Unfairly accusing oneself or others of the occasion.

- Inability to feel positive feelings like joy and fulfilment

- Lack of enthusiasm for recently delighted in exercises

- Feeling disconnected from others.

Most instances of PTSD start inside the initial three months after the trauma.

However, a few people may not create side effects until a half year or later.

<u>HISTORY OF PTSD</u>

Before current medication, specialists thought posttraumatic stress was a physical condition. American Civil War records talk about a condition called "Da Costa's Syndrome." Soldiers determined to have the disorder would have Anxiety, a quick heartbeat, and inconvenience relaxing. Surgeons expected the warriors had overstimulated their hearts. Officers got medication to control their side effects and came back to war before long. In World War I, posttraumatic stress was designated "shell stun." Common side effects of shell stun included cerebral pains, flashbacks, and affectability to noisy commotions. Doctors thought warriors' manifestations were because of brain harm from big guns shells. Yet, numerous warriors who hadn't been close to blasts demonstrated shell stun also. Researchers expelled this subsequent gathering as having "a shortcoming of nerves."

Present-day investigate shows no connection between PTSD and versatility. There is no proof that people with PTSD are genuinely flimsier than any other individual. In any case, in the mid-twentieth century, fighters with posttraumatic stress frequently confronted extraordinary shame. During WWI and WWII, the military's need was generally returning warriors to the front line as opposed to advancing psychological wellness. The DSM didn't list posttraumatic stress as a finding until 1980. By at that point, researchers had information from Vietnam veterans, Holocaust survivors, and more. Specialists concurred PTSD was a psychological well-being condition instead of physical damage or character imperfection.

PTSD IN MODERN VETERANS

Because of the idea of the current fighting, veterans from Iraq and Afghanistan are particularly prone to confront trauma. The U.S. Division gauges 10-18% of veterans create PTSD after they return. An officer's danger of PTSD relies upon their socioeconomics and their encounters in battle.

Warriors who are unmarried and have lower levels of instruction are bound to have PTSD. Female help individuals likewise have more severe dangers of PTSD. As indicated by a recent report, 5% of female troopers revealed rape. In the military, ladies are multiple times bound to encounter rape than men. Warriors who face more battle stressors are bound to create PTSD. Battle stressors incorporate seeing bodies, having a companion slaughtered, being trapped, and getting harmed in a fight. Fighters with more extended arrangement periods additionally had higher paces of posttraumatic stress.

PTSD AND GENDER

In America, ladies are more than twice as likely as men to create PTSD. An expected 9.7% of ladies will encounter PTSD in their lifetimes, contrasted with 3.6 % of men. The distinction might be mostly because of how ladies experience higher paces of rape and abusive behavior at home. Assault is one of the traumas well on the way to prompt posttraumatic stress (Others incorporate military battle, politically-propelled internment, and decimation.).

PTSD IN RACIAL AND ETHNIC MINORITIES

Some racial and ethnic minorities have higher paces of posttraumatic stress. A 2011 investigation of the general U.S. populace found the most elevated pace of PTSD among dark occupants (8.7%). White people had a lifetime commonness of 7.4%, and Hispanic occupants had a pace of 7.0%. Asians had the most minimal paces of PTSD (4.0%).

Specific minority subgroups additionally have higher PTSD rates. A few assessments propose that the portion of Holocaust survivors have posttraumatic stress. In any case, ethnic and racial commonness rates change between thinks about. How an investigation characterizes PTSD or which individuals it remembers for a minority gathering can influence information. A few analyses have discovered higher paces of PTSD among Hispanic Americans than either dark or white Americans.

A PTSD finding requires an individual to have encountered trauma. Contrasts in trauma presentation may assume an enormous job in racial and ethnic PTSD rates. Racial and ethnic minorities frequently face various traumas from different gatherings. These traumas may include:

- Racism and segregation: Prejudice can cause distress and negative life results. For example, enlisting segregation can prompt joblessness.

- Exposure to savagery: Minorities might be presented to wars, ethnic and racialized viciousness, and wrongdoing. Viciousness by military or law requirement officials can likewise be a hazard.

An analysis distributed in 2010 contends current PTSD measures may neglect to represent the traumas of bigotry and ethnoviolence. Vicarious trauma, for example, watching police viciousness on TV, may go about as an impetus for PTSD. Although the individual sitting in front of the TV isn't in direct peril, they might be helped to remember authentic dangers to their character gathering. Since despise wrongdoings are frequently coordinated toward a gathering, an individual may feel focused on. Research recommends PTSD might be under-analyzed in some minority gatherings. A recent report overviewed African-Americans with a trauma history.

Generally, 50% of the members didn't talk about their history or indications with a human services supplier. At the point when individuals shared their side effects, they were more averse to be determined to have PTSD. Different analysis bolsters the possibility that racial and ethnic minorities are less inclined to get treatment for posttraumatic stress.

MULTIFACETED COMPARISON OF PTSD RATES

Estimating multifaceted PTSD rates can be troublesome. Most PTSD investigate has concentrated on individuals living in Western countries. In any event, when scientists survey PTSD rates in non-Western countries, social contrasts can make it challenging to think about outcomes. Yet, the exploration accessible so far proposes PTSD rates do change crosswise over societies.

A recent report looked at PTSD rates between individuals living in different European countries. The analysis found the most noteworthy rate (6.67%) among Croatians. Human qualities were a more prominent indicator of PTSD rates than trauma presentation. Sensation-chasing was firmly connected to PTSD rates.

An individual's danger of trauma introduction relies upon numerous social components, including:

- Where they live

- Their social class inside that culture

- How much network bolster they have

- Political strife

Excellent presentation to viciousness regularly corresponds to a high pace of PTSD. Displaced people are more probable than non-outcasts to create PTSD. The World Health Organization gauges 1% of non-outcasts have the condition. By correlation, numerous investigations have set the predominance rate among outcasts at 15%. The most significant research survey to date included exiles from 40 unique countries. This audit gauges 30% of outcasts has PTSD.

<u>PTSD IN CHILDREN</u>

Kids can create posttraumatic stress along these lines to grown-ups. Be that as it may, there are a couple of side effects one of a kind to kids. Youngsters 12 and more youthful commonly don't have flashbacks how grown-ups do. However, it is normal for youngsters to reenact the trauma through play. For example, a youngster who saw a school shooting may more than once play with imagining weapons. Kids with PTSD may accept there were notice signs before the traumatic occasion. They may look for these signs so they can "anticipate" the next event.

Young people with PTSD frequently creates pessimistic convictions about themselves. They may pass judgment on themselves as "harmed" or "fearful" contrasted with their friends. They may likewise demonstrate hesitance to attempt age-fitting exercises like driving or dating. Youths with PTSD are bound to create hatred and hazard taking practices than individuals of different ages.

PTSD AND CO-OCCURRING MENTAL HEALTH CONDITIONS

Individuals with PTSD are 80% bound to have a comorbid psychological well-being worry than those without the condition. Depression, substance misuse, and uneasiness regularly co-happen with PTSD. Youngsters with PTSD are probably going to have comorbid oppositional disobedient conduct and partition Anxiety. Veterans with PTSD are 48% prone likewise to have mellow traumatic brain damage. Other psychological well-being issues can fuel PTSD side effects. They may bring down the state of mind, upset focus, or bring out forceful propensities. These confusing issues can keep people from looking for help. They may confine themselves from friends and family or stay away from treatment assets. If somebody with PTSD has a comorbid condition, it very well may be tough for them to get important consideration.

A therapist can distinguish if co-happening conditions are adding to PTSD. Therapy can help somebody diminish indications from PTSD and some other analyses. There is no disgrace in looking for help.

<u>FINDING SUPPORT FOR POSTTRAUMATIC STRESS</u>

Recuperation from posttraumatic stress (PTSD) is a voyage that takes an alternate shape for every person. It is rarely too soon or past the point where it is possible to look for psychotherapy. Medications can help individuals beat indications and proceed onward from posttraumatic stress through and through. As per trauma therapist "We may maintain a strategic distance from circumstances or individuals that help us to remember the trauma. We might be genuinely numb, discouraged, or anxious...If you experience such sentiments, musings, or practices after a trauma, realize that such encounters are human and nothing to be embarrassed about. Through the help of a prepared proficient, one can mend from the results of trauma."

THERAPY FOR POSTTRAUMATIC STRESS

Therapy frequently helps individuals understand their encounters. Advising won't delete the trauma, yet it can relieve difficult emotions from that trauma. A therapist can instruct solid, adapting aptitudes to decrease the seriousness and recurrence of side effects. Therapy can manage an individual to posttraumatic development, reaffirming their inward quality.

There are many proof-based medicines for PTSD. A portion of the more typical modalities include:

- Eye development desensitization and reprocessing (EMDR): This methodology was explicitly intended to treat PTSD. A therapist will utilize tangible prompts to help individuals process traumatic recollections.

- Exposure therapy: This treatment opens a person to tokens of the trauma in a protected space. A therapist can help the individual with any distress that outcomes. In a perfect world, an individual will develop desensitized to the memory over rehashed sessions.

- Cognitive processing therapy (CPT): A type of intellectual conduct therapy utilized explicitly for trauma. An individual can figure out how trauma has influenced their convictions and how these contemplations thusly influence conduct. CPT can help people break destructive examples of cynicism.

- Logotherapy: This treatment tends to an individual's existential worries after trauma. It can help somebody discover importance after loss.

- Group therapy: A prepared therapist will control a gathering of 4-12 individuals in exchange. Gathering therapy can give social help to individuals who may somehow or another separate themselves.

Sometimes, psychotropic medicine might be utilized in blend with therapy. Individuals with PTSD may discover prescription helpful for improving rest and settling the state of mind. The vast majority with PTSD who get therapy can recoup. On the off chance that somebody is as yet battling in spite of treatment, they may have a co-happening analysis. Conditions, for example, depression can meddle with treatment when they go unacknowledged. Regardless of whether an individual came to therapy for PTSD explicitly, it is frequently helpful to treat analyze in tandem.

HELP FOR LOVED ONES OF PEOPLE WITH PTSD

Individuals whose friends and family have PTSD may battle to decide how they can help. Once in a while, the person with PTSD realizes what they need most. They may request help with everyday errands. They may require exhortation. They may need somebody to tune in to their story without judgment. Loved ones might have the option to offer these things. Be that as it may, a few people may attempt to help and wind up being harmed themselves. One normal test is vicarious trauma. Hearing somebody talk about a traumatic encounter can cause passionate distress and weariness. Aberrant introduction to traumas, for example, assault or military battle would itself be able to be traumatic. Individuals who give progressing care to a friend or family member with PTSD may experience the ill effects of parental figure stress. Numerous guardians experience emotional well-being issues, for example, depression and uneasiness. Now and again, a guardian might be presented to trauma (optional or direct) and create PTSD themselves.

Therapy can help with these difficulties. A parental figure can likewise profit by self-care methodologies, for example,

- Talking to a steady companion

- Taking time away from providing care

- Setting clear limits with a consideration beneficiary who may have irrational desires.

Loved ones are probably not going to fix a friend or family member of PTSD. At the point when a friend or family member has posttraumatic stress, they likely need psychological well-being proficient.

A therapist has the preparation required to survey an individual's indications. They can decide the proper treatment for an individual's circumstance. If mate or relative has been influenced by a friend or family member's PTSD, they may profit by joint directing.

COMPLEMENTARY AND ALTERNATIVE MEDICINE FOR PTSD

Numerous individuals with PTSD utilize complementary and alternative medicine (CAM). CAMs are medications set outside of traditional Western medicine, for example, yoga or aromatherapy. They are used regularly in tandem with standard consideration.

The Department of Veterans Affairs (VA) says CAM use is particularly necessary among veterans with PTSD. A 2012 overview discovered 39% of veterans with PTSD had utilized CAM in the earlier year. Another investigation indicated veterans with PTSD were 25% bound to use CAM than their friends without PTSD. Ninety-six percent of the VA's treatment programs for PTSD offer at any rate one CAM treatment.

As indicated by the VA, the proof is blended concerning the viability of CAM. Needle therapy has the most evidence of profiting individuals with PTSD. Contemplation and dynamic unwinding strategies likewise show unassuming advantages. As a rule, specialists don't suggest utilizing CAM as a substitution for proof-based medications. However, CAM can be a decent supplement to therapy and drug. Emotional well-being proficient can help people pick which CAMs best fit their needs.

CASE EXAMPLES OF THERAPY FOR PTSD

- **Iraq war veteran thinks that its hard to straighten out to regular citizen life:** Ricky, 26, has as of late come back from Iraq, where she saw substantial battle. She discloses to her therapist she was fine until the prior week. A burglary had happened in a nearby store while she was there. All of a sudden, Ricky was deadened by realistic recollections of her time in battle. From that point forward, she has had nightmares about Iraq blended in with pictures of her home. Ricky feels overpowered and on edge about these flashbacks. She additionally has some blame related with not halting the neighborhood burglary, having disguised demonstrations of grit as her obligation and duty. In therapy, Ricky investigates her convictions about being a veteran and what she anticipates from herself. The therapist shows Ricky some unwinding and establishing exercises. At Ricky's solicitation, the therapist offers a mental referral against nervousness medicine to help Ricky rest. Ricky chooses to join a therapy bunch for veterans who experience related issues. A year after her first visit, she is never again taking prescription. Ricky is feeling increasingly cheerful; however regardless, she battles with extraordinary pain about the war.

- **Repercussions of youth misuse**: Pat, 52, looks for therapy for help with his nervousness. His history uncovers severe physical maltreatment as a kid, which Pat is hesitant to return to. Pat's therapist doesn't drive him to return to the occasions yet delicately brings the maltreatment up in a later session. At the point when she does, Pat turns out to be disturbed. In the following session, the therapist welcomes Pat to analyze his irate reaction. Pat concurs that his response shows the maltreatment is as yet influencing him. Pat's therapist suggests eye development desensitization and reprocessing (EMDR) therapy. He starts EMDR sessions, which help him recognize the maltreatment in a generally possible manner. After a few sessions, Pat can defy his harsh past more straightforwardly and mend from it. His nervousness levels reduce after some time.

POSTTRAUMATIC GROWTH

The healing adventure after a traumatic occasion, for example, misuse, abusive behavior at home, military battle, loss, or different kinds of mental change will probably appear to be unique for every individual. The advancement toward more noteworthy psychological wellness and passionate prosperity, a period during which an individual may be partaking in psychotherapy and different kinds of treatment, can be called posttraumatic development. Therapists Richard Tedeschi, PhD, and Lawrence Calhoun, PhD, built up the theory of posttraumatic development during the 1990s. Although recouping from the impacts of trauma was not new, the presentation of posttraumatic development developed as a systematic report in brain research, social work, science, and advising in light of

Tedeschi's and Calhoun's impact. Today, it is an idea numerous therapist use to help move individuals in therapy toward constructive change, evaluate the advancement of individuals healing from trauma, and better understand the change procedure as somebody recuperates.

WHAT IS POSTTRAUMATIC GROWTH?

At its generally oversimplified, posttraumatic development is specific to change that can occur for an individual after encountering trauma or a significant life emergency. The procedure may be distinctive dependent on the sort of trauma an individual suffered, what sorts of therapy the individual encounters subsequently, and the degrees of help they can rely upon all through treatment. As the opposite of posttraumatic stress or PTSD, posttraumatic development can be portrayed by the signs one is beating the hurtful impacts of trauma. A few therapists have depicted posttraumatic development as synonymous with flexibility. Yet, while strength infers a capacity to bob back after trauma, posttraumatic development recognises an individual's ceaseless, now and then long-lasting, endeavours to move past trauma and the impacts of PTSD. Putting an accentuation on the posttraumatic event can help center the remedial procedure on somebody's endurance after trauma, however their capacity to flourish.

<u>WHAT DOES POSTTRAUMATIC GROWTH RESEMBLE?</u>

Therapists utilize different appraisal instruments to gauge the manners by which an individual has accomplished development after trauma. One technique created by Tedeschi and Calhoun is known as the Posttraumatic Growth Inventory (PTGI). In this model, psychological wellness experts utilize five zones to survey for positive change:

- Appreciation of life

- Relationships with others

- New potential outcomes throughout everyday life

- Personal quality

- Spiritual change

This format for posttraumatic development isn't widespread, and there are numerous ways it may move by a person. For instance, Tedeschi and Calhoun keep on altering the marker of otherworldly change given this factor doesn't generally have an impact in individuals' recuperation travels and may appear to be unique dependent on somebody's social foundation.

As opposed to depending alone translations of somebody's development through the treatment procedure, psychological wellness experts utilize self-reports from individuals in therapy to gauge accomplishments and achievements in healing. Furthermore, these markers for development can offer progressively explicit goals for the individual in therapy–an opportunity to concentrate on singular parts of one's life, instead of a shapeless thought of what positive change implies.

WHAT CONTRIBUTES TO POSTTRAUMATIC GROWTH?

Having the ceaseless, dependable inclusion of a psychotherapist commonly helps help the procedure of posttraumatic development. Not exclusively can therapists extensively survey how trauma has influenced an individual and what parts of PTSD they might be encountering; they can likewise manage the recuperation procedure such that offers expectation and consolation. Seeing a therapist after trauma requires some responsibility and resolve–both fundamental components of posttraumatic development.

Notwithstanding therapy, Calhoun and Tedeschi refer to a tight close to a supportive home group of people, idealism, and local gatherings as variables that can help somebody advance toward posttraumatic development. A few components may make an individual increasingly inclined to posttraumatic development. These incorporate sex (ladies are statistically bound to encounter posttraumatic event), the nonappearance of various traumatic scenes from quite a while ago, and now and again, raised financial status.

In any case, scientists keep up posttraumatic development is feasible for anybody. Now and again, even outside impacts that would appear to be boundaries to healing have demonstrated compelling. For instance, somebody in trauma recuperation may encounter a loss that makes them assume greater responsibility for their life and feel much more grounded. And more established trauma survivors might be bound to set aside some effort to sustain familial bonds or close connections, as opposed to pushing ahead into diverting their lives.

USEFUL EFFECTS OF POSTTRAUMATIC GROWTH

Trauma can have an extensive negative impact on practically any part of one's life. Physical, mental, and passionate wellbeing are all in danger when one encounters an actual existence emergency, savagery, misuse, or enthusiastic change. Healing from these encounters, in whatever structure that takes, is probably going to affect all parts of a person's life decidedly.

Posttraumatic development can increase significantly less the side effects of PTSD, for example, mental trips, nightmares, flashbacks, Anxiety, and depression. It might likewise help address physical parts of posttraumatic stress, as PTSD has been connected to cardiovascular infection, constant weakness, diabetes, gastrointestinal issues, and more.

Since trauma, PTSD, and co-happening emotional wellness issues like substance misuse and depression would all be able to have a substantial unfavorable impact on prosperity, any advancement toward checking these are probably going to be helpful. Posttraumatic development can help improve one's enthusiastic wellbeing, mental prosperity, and physical health after trauma.

CHAPTER SIX

UNDERSTANDING ANXIETY

In this segment, we need to get further under the skin of 'anxiety', one of our most unwelcomed passionate states, and understand the job that it plays in our lives—for better and in negative ways. It isn't our plan to show the case for killing anxiety, for being restless is a significant piece of being human. We are often nervous about those parts of our lives that we generally care about: our wellbeing; our capacity to dress and bolster ourselves and our family; and our capacity to be associated and esteemed by others. Anxiety helps us to get up toward the beginning of the day and inspires us to step out of our customary range of familiarity. Be that as it may, we often put everything on the line to abstain from being restless, feeling a feeling of disappointment on the off chance that we don't hold our stressing contemplations under tight control. There might be times when these musings escape from us and start to feel overpowering. For some they may get routine, prompting normal awkward, or in any event, distressing, physical side effects. Examples of evasion may develop, that can limitingly affect our lives. Anxiety can likewise be elating. Placing ourselves into circumstances that make us restless can feel like a trial at the time, however breaking through to the opposite side can bring an incredible feeling of accomplishment. Our most significant minutes in life are typically not accomplished without some restless evenings. Being another parent, our wedding days, breezing through tests and figuring out how to drive bring incredible prizes, yet it is improbable that these were accomplished without particular sentiments of dread. Anxiety is a passionate expression that can work for us just as against us. It is something we as a whole share for all intents and purpose; however, where we often vary is by the way we see these sentiments of excitement and how we react to them. Our life conditions, our childhood and our characters would all be able to be factored in why one individual's energizing carnival ride will leave someone else in contemptible fear. Feeling on edge is anything but an indication of disappointment, and there are times when it is critical to request help from everyone around us, or from professionals. Notwithstanding, as we come to understand anxiety better, there is a lot of that we can do as people to find a way to decrease its hold over us and to figure out how to value our full scope of feelings unafraid that they will surpass us.

WHAT IS ANXIETY?

Everybody has sentiments of anxiety sooner or later in their life, regardless of whether it is tied in with the planning for a prospective employee meet-up, meeting an accomplice's family just because, or the possibility of parenthood. While we partner anxiety with modifications to our mental state, experienced as stress or fear may be, and physical side effects, for example, raised pulse and adrenaline, we likewise understand that it is probably going to influence us just briefly until the wellspring of our anxiety has passed or we have figured out how to adapt to it. Anxiety is in this manner one of a scope of feelings that serves the positive capacity of cautioning us to things we may need to stress over: conceivably destructive things. All the more significantly, these feelings help us to assess potential dangers and suitably react to them, maybe by enlivening our reflexes or concentrating. Dread, similar to anxiety, is a recognizable feeling definitely because it is a piece of everybody's understanding, and we think of it as a fundamental segment of our humankind. Yet, it is likewise a mental, physiological and social state we share with creatures when faced by a danger to our prosperity or endurance. Dread expands the body's excitement, anticipation, and neurobiological action, and triggers specific standards of conduct intended to help us adapt to an unfavorable or surprising circumstance. In any case, how would we recognize anxiety from dread, given that the two are often utilized reciprocally?

While dread often has a particular, prompt setting which incites great 'fight or flight' reflexes—the programmed dread reaction happens quicker than cognizant idea, discharging floods of adrenaline which can die down rapidly once the apparent or real danger has passed—anxiety implies waiting for fear, an interminable feeling of stress, strain or fear, the wellsprings of which might be indistinct. It very well may be a dubious, unsavory feeling experienced fully expecting some not well-characterized adversity. The council accused of inspecting the diagnostic criteria for the most recent variant of the

Diagnostic and Statistical Manual of Mental Disorders (DSM) correspondingly recognize anxiety as "a future-situated temperament state related with groundwork for conceivable, up and coming negative occasions" from dread which "is an alert reaction to present or inevitable peril (genuine or saw)"; however include "critically, these portrayals speak to models of dread and anxiety that lie at better places upon a continuum of reacting. Along such a continuum, indications of dread versus anxiety are probably going to wander and unite to changing degrees. Another essayist, communicating the differentiation in less elusive terms, proposes "the abrupt re-game plan of your guts when a gatecrasher holds a blade to your back (dread), is unique concerning the gentle sickness, discombobulation and butterflies in your stomach as you're going to make a troublesome telephone call (anxiety)." This report is worried about the way that various sorts of anxiety, found at different focuses on the continuum, are experienced by people and how they are spoken to the more extensive open. It investigates the common indications just as what happens when anxiety turns out to be more than a brief encounter and instead is experienced as either a progression of incapacitating scenes or a consistent nearness in somebody's life. Anxiety disorders, for example, frenzy, fears and fanatical practices might be activated by traumatic recollections, nonsensical contempt of specific items, closeness to particular circumstances or physical areas, or industrious stress that something terrible will occur later on. A characterizing normal for anxiety disorders is that mental indications, for example, fractiousness, challenges concentrating and depression, become steady and meddling. Numerous individuals likewise experience physical manifestations, similar to heart palpitations, perspiring, pressures and torment, substantial and quick breathing, discombobulation, swooning, heartburn, stomach hurts, disorder and loose bowels; in severe cases, individuals have portrayed how it felt just as they were passing on. The lives of those with the most extreme types of anxiety can turn out to be ruled by their condition, which means they think that it's hard to unwind or accomplish ordinary examples of rest, getting stuck in round examples of imagined that debilitate their capacity to keep up favored ways of life, hold down work or continue individual relationships. Anxiety can mean nervousness, stress, or self-question. Here and there, the reason for uneasiness is anything but difficult to spot, while different occasions it may not be. Everybody feels some degree of nervousness on occasion. In any case, overpowering, repeating, or "out of the blue" fear can profoundly affect individuals. At the point when nervousness meddles this way, conversing with a therapist can help.

ANXIETY AND MODERNITY

Although it is the most well-known indication of mental distress in almost every nation on the planet, anxiety is often introduced as a relic of current Western social orders; Norman Mailer, for instance, proposed that "the regular job of twentieth-century man [sic] is anxiety". The idea of anxiety, in essence, was first brought to conspicuousness as a philosophical and psychoanalytic idea in the initial segment of the twentieth century. Freud was a major figure in the advancement of Western considering anxiety, which he thought about as a condition of inward pressure from which people are headed to getaway. At an essential level, anxiety is a sign to the sense of self (the part of the character that manages reality) that something overwhelmingly terrible is going to occur and that it needs to utilize a guard instrument accordingly. Freud considered this to be getting from a newborn child's mental helplessness, which is a partner of its natural helplessness. People figure out how to adapt to anxiety incited by 'gcnuine' dangers, for example, the dread of being chewed by a canine, either by keeping away from circumstances prone to contain the risk or by physically pulling back from them. Freud's typology likewise included masochist anxiety emerging from an oblivious dread that we will lose control of libidinal motivations, prompting improper conduct, and good anxiety, emerging from dread of abusing our good or cultural codes. Moral anxiety, he recommended, shows itself as blame or disgrace. The assignment of analysis is along these lines to fortify the capacity of the self-image to discover methods for adapting to anxiety, for example, 'disavowal', 'defense', 'relapse' (to a youth state) or 'projection'. Inside the existentialist philosophical custom, 'apprehension', from the German word for anxiety, is held to be a negative inclination emerging from the experience of human opportunity and obligation in this present reality where confidence and conventional social bonds have been undermined. Kierkegaard's exemplary case of existential apprehension is of an individual standing on the edge of a high bluff or working; alongside the dread of incidentally falling, the individual feels a nonsensical motivation to throw themselves over the edge purposely. The feeling the individual feels after understanding that the person has this alternative is tension. Kierkegaard depicted the weight of settling on moral decisions as a result of through and through freedom "the tipsiness of opportunity". Existential brain science along these lines continues from the assumption that anxiety originates from an emergency in the exercise of through and through freedom, which may be showed in anxiety about one's mortality, the certainty of loss, or about tolerating moral duty regarding one's considerations, emotions and activities. That anxiety "some way or another feels new" might be clarified somewhat by the way that anxiety has been the subject of noteworthy logical research for not exactly 50 years, while the mental profession previously arranged diagnostic criteria for all the various disorders as of late as 1980, with the distribution of DSM-III. Resulting propels in diagnostic methods, combined with the improvement of successful pharmacological medicines and mental treatments, have provoked essential human services professionals to all the more promptly distinguish anxiety in their patients. Anxiety is currently perceived as one of the most pervasive mental medical issues in the UK. Yet, there is great proof that it is still underreported, under-analyzed and under-treated. One explanation might be that, not normal for some other mental medical problems, individuals whose lives are influenced have not yet discovered a voice that verbalizes the full scope of encounters of anxiety, not only those of individuals living with anxiety disorders. As of late, this has started to change, as authors, bloggers and campaigners have furnished us with a knowledge into "England's quiet plague" by depicting the lived understanding of anxiety, the complexities and subtleties of the different disorders, the indications that are related with them, and the impact that anxiety has upon their lives. For instance, a few people living with anxiety portray sentiments of disgrace and shame at their physical indications, for example, unnecessary sweat, which lead them to embrace what Freudian psychoanalysts would perceive as old-style guard systems: "they figure out how to close their anxiety from general visibility". As per Daniel Smith, "they figure out how to plug their anxiety inside themselves like corrosive in a vial. It isn't charming. The human personality isn't Pyrex; it can consume. In any case, it works." Perhaps more altogether, the declaration of individuals living with anxiety bears us an increasingly adjusted energy about the job that it plays in molding their lives; as Scott Stossel, creator of My Age of Anxiety, puts it, "anxiety can be a spike to accomplishment just as a hindrance. Picture a ringer bend with extraordinary anxiety on the extreme right and excessive absence of anxiety on the extreme left. In case you're excessively on edge to where it's physically and mentally crippling, at that point your exhibition endures. In case you're not on edge enough, on the off chance that you're not locked in and marginally initiated by anxiety, so to speak, at that point your exhibition additionally endures." The voices of individuals living with the more intense types of anxiety help us to imagine anxiety as something more than essentially a condition that requires conclusion and treatment. How people draw in with their anxiety, how they oversee it and speak to it to the more extensive world lifts anxiety past the domain of medicine and science and into a more extensive sociological and social setting.

WHAT ARE THE MOST WELL-KNOWN ANXIETY DISORDERS?

The experience of anxiety often includes a heap of interconnected side effects and disorders portrayed by befuddling circularity between the triggers to

anxiety and the reactions that it conjures.
Scott Stossel's "pack" incorporates
emetophobia, a dread of retching
(particularly out in the open), which is a
condition that as per Anxiety UK isn't
broadly analyzed even though it is
genuinely predominant. This is the part
of his anxiety that is generally
weakening, he says, since it is laced with
agoraphobia caused explicitly by a dread
of being debilitated a long way from
home just as sickness, an ordinarily
experienced physical manifestation of
numerous types of anxiety. While the
different components to the group may
not, in themselves, decisively affect his

life, the impacts of their association can be destroying. This can be seen all the more obvious in individuals determined to have co-dismal depression and anxiety, which often results from a downward winding in which anxiety prompts low mindset, which thusly heightens the anxiety. The latest national review of mental wellbeing in the UK demonstrates that while 2.6% of the populace experience depression and 4.7% have anxiety issues, the same number of as 9.7% endure blended depression and anxiety, making it the most predominant mental medical issue among the populace overall. Past reviews led in 1993 and 2000 demonstrated an expansion in the pervasiveness of blended anxiety and burdensome disorders, yet just little changes somewhere in the range of 2000 and 2007.

Panic is a distortion of the body's ordinary reaction to dread, stress or fervor. Fits of anxiety are a time of extraordinary dread wherein manifestations grow unexpectedly and top quickly. Fits of anxiety have been depicted as a type of "enthusiastic short-circuiting" whereby the limbic brain all of a sudden assumes control over the body's working, prompting overpowering sensations, which may incorporate a beating heart, feeling faint, perspiring, flimsy appendages, sickness, chest torments, breathing uneasiness and sentiments of losing control. Adrenaline overpowers the psychological capacities that would typically help the brain survey the genuine idea of the danger to the body. The impacts can be extreme to the point that individuals encountering alarm assaults accepted they were kicking the bucket. It is evaluated that 1.2% of the UK populace experience alarm as a different issue, ascending to

1.7% for those encountering it with agoraphobia.

Fear is an extreme and unreasonable dread of a particular item or circumstance, with the end goal that it urges the individual to encounter it to try hard to maintain a strategic distance from it. Fears can be about unsafe things or circumstances that present a hazard; however, they can likewise be of innocuous circumstances, objects or now and then creatures. Social fear can incorporate a dread of being judged, investigated or embarrassed somehow or another. It can show itself with a dread of doing certain things before others, for example, open talking. As indicated by the Office for National Statistics, around 1.9% of British grown-ups experience a fear of some depiction, and ladies are twice as likely as men to be influenced by this issue.

Although agoraphobia is often connected with a dread of open spaces, the principle include is extreme anxiety setting off a frenzy reaction in circumstances where getaway is seen as troublesome or conceivably humiliating, or where help may not be promptly accessible; in fact, such emergencies often happen in restricted spaces. Individuals with agoraphobia seem to encounter two unmistakable kinds of anxiety— alarm, and the anticipatory anxiety identified with dread of future fits of anxiety. Agoraphobia can have an emotional restricting impact upon the way of life of individuals living with the condition, as they try to maintain a strategic distance from circumstances that make them on edge; for instance, just utilizing spots where leave courses are known or remaining nearby to exits. In outrageous cases, people are so dreadful they become homebound inside and out. Beginning of agoraphobia is for the most part between the ages of 18 and 35 and influences somewhere in the range of 1.5% and 3.5% of the overall public in its entirely created structure; in a less severe structure up to one of every eight individuals, for example around 7 million in the UK, might be upset by some agoraphobic side effects.

Post-Traumatic Stress Disorder (PTSD), or disorder, is a mental response to an exceptionally stressful occasion outside the scope of ordinary experience, for example, military battle, physical brutality, or a cataclysmic event. The manifestations, for the most part, incorporate depression, anxiety, flashbacks, intermittent nightmares, and shirking of circumstances that may trigger recollections of the occasion. One investigation of UK military workforce sent to Afghanistan found that of 1,431 members, 2.7% were named having likely PTSD. At the same time, a family unit overview of UK grown-ups assessed a commonness of 2.6% in men and 3.3% in ladies. While the scope of studies researching the wellbeing difficulties of shelter searchers and displaced people have discovered that PTSD levels can be as much as multiple times higher than the age-coordinated overall public. A scope of stressors has been distinguished as affecting antagonistically on mental wellbeing, including that accomplished premigration, for example, torment, traumatic deprivation and detainment, yet in addition post-relocation factors, for example, separation, confinement, dejection and deferred basic leadership in the shelter procedure. One investigation of ladies' refuge searchers in Scotland, and Belgium found that 57% were over the cut-point for PTSD symptomatology.

Obsessive-Compulsive Disorder (OCD) influences around 2 3% of the populace.

It is described by undesirable, meddlesome, diligent or tedious musings, emotions, thoughts, sensations (fixations), or practices that make the sufferer feel headed to accomplish something (impulses) to dispose of the obsessive considerations. This gives transitory alleviation and not playing out the obsessive customs can cause incredible anxiety. An individual's degree of OCD can be anyplace from mellow to extreme, however on the off chance that severe and left untreated; it can crush an individual's ability to work at work, at school or even to lead an agreeable presence in the home.

Generalized Anxiety Disorder (GAD) is the most ordinarily analyzed anxiety disorder and as a rule influences youthful grown-up. Ladies are bound to be influenced than men. While sentiments of anxiety are ordinary, individuals with GAD think that its difficult to control them, to such a degree, that it infringes upon their day by day life. It makes sufferers feel on edge about a wide scope of circumstances and issues, instead of one explicit occasion. In contrast to a fear, which centers upon a particular book or circumstance, summed up anxiety is diffuse and overruns the sufferer's day by day life. Although GAD is less severe than a fit of anxiety, its length and the mental and physical side effects, for example, crabbiness, poor fixation and the impacts of disturbed rest designs, imply that individuals with the disorder often think that it is hard to carry on with the existence they would want to live. Stray influences 2–5% of the populace and has expanded somewhat since 1993, yet represents as much as 30% of the mental medical issues in individuals seen by GPs, which clarifies why an analysis of individuals looking for help through essential consideration recommends a higher commonness pace of 7.2%.

<u>ANXIETY AND WELLBEING</u>

The genuine effect of anxiety can be covered when it is the manifestation of other increasingly evident or treatable physical issues which are probably going to be organized in any consequent therapeutic mediation. Anxiety issues are regular among cardiovascular patients; for instance, alarm disorder is up to multiple times increasingly common among individuals with interminable obstructive pneumonic sickness than in the overall public

Individuals with GAD have been seen as a greater danger of coronary illness. In contrast, anxiety has likewise been connected to the expanded occurrence of gastrointestinal issues, joint pain, headaches, sensitivities, and thyroid infection. Individuals with anxiety disorders are multiple times as likely as others to grow hypertension, and numerous investigations have indicated a connection among anxiety and decreased white blood cell work, an indication of resistant system shortcoming. There is likewise developing proof of a connection between stress and Alzheimer's illness. Anxiety is additionally connected with an unfortunate way of life decisions, for example, smoking, drinking a lot of liquor, and a horrible eating routine.

SIGNS AND SYMPTOMS OF ANXIETY

Diagnosing uneasiness relies upon an individual's sentiments of stress so that manifestations will change. Character, co-happening emotional well-being conditions, and different variables may clarify an individual's side effects.

Anxiety can cause meddlesome or over the top contemplations. An individual with anxiety may feel bewildered or think that it's difficult to focus. Feeling fretful or baffled can likewise be an indication of uneasiness. Others with nervousness may feel discouraged.

Side effects of Anxiety can likewise be physical. Nervousness can cause excessively tense muscles or hyper Anxiety. Trembling, perspiring, a dashing heartbeat, discombobulation, and a sleeping disorder can also originate from Anxiety. Anxiety may even cause migraines, stomach related issues, trouble breathing, and sickness. On the off chance that physical manifestations of uneasiness are severe and unexpected, it might be a fit of anxiety.

WHAT DOES ANXIETY RESEMBLE?

Individuals can give indications of uneasiness from numerous points of view. Some may turn out to be increasingly talkative, while others pull back or self-detach. Indeed, even individuals who appear to be cordial, agreeable, or brave can have Anxiety. Since Anxiety has numerous manifestations, what it looks like for one individual isn't the way it shows up for another.

Individuals who have nervousness might be pulled back; however, this isn't the situation for everybody with uneasiness. Now and then, uneasiness may trigger a "fight" instead of "flight" reaction, in which case an individual may seem angry. Bumbling over words, trembling, and nervous tics are regularly connected with nervousness. While they can show up in individuals with Anxiety, they are not always present, and a few people who don't have nervousness additionally give these indications.

On the off chance that you are uncertain on the off chance that somebody you know might be encountering nervousness, it may not be helpful to bring it up except if they do. Be that as it may, there are a few moves you can consider making on the off chance that you need to make an individual who may be on edge increasingly agreeable. You can:

- Be quiet with them

- Share inspirational statements or appreciation.

- Be unsurprising and be eager to impart subtleties to them if they inquire.

WHAT DOES GENERALIZED ANXIETY MEAN?

Generalized Anxiety is otherwise called free-drifting Anxiety. It is recognized by ceaseless sentiments of fate and stress that have no immediate reason. Numerous individuals feel on edge about specific things, similar to cash, prospective employee meet-ups, or dating. However, individuals with free-coasting Anxiety can feel on edge for no unmistakable explanation. Generalized Anxiety can likewise mean inclination an excess of stress over a specific occasion.

The Diagnostic and Statistical Manual (DSM-5) distinguishes generalized anxiety disorder (GAD) as over the top stress that affects an individual on a practically everyday schedule. It should be most recent a half year or more and be hard to control. It should likewise not have the option to be better clarified by some other wellbeing condition. An individual determined to have GAD should also appear in any event three of the accompanying side effects:

- Frequent weakness

- Restlessness

- Irritability

- Difficulty centring

- Sleep issues

- Muscle strain

Numerous elements can add to free-coasting nervousness. Living in stressful or harsh situations might be a reason. In some cases, nervousness turns into a propensity. An individual used to feeling on edge about an occasion may continue feeling on edge once it is finished. A few therapists fight that advanced life causes free-coasting nervousness. As indicated by them, cutoff times, quick-paced ways of life, and staying aware of social media could create interminable Anxiety.

At the point when an individual can't discover where their anxiety originates from, therapy can help. Therapy regularly helps individuals get the hang of adapting abilities for managing side effects of stress. Aptitudes that help individuals with constant anxiety incorporate profound breathing, reflection, exercise, and individual correspondence.

WHAT CAUSES ANXIETY?

Anxiety, similar to the fight, flight, or freeze reaction, is for endurance. It enables individuals to secure themselves to evade hurt. Once in a while, an individual has elevated levels of anxiety routinely. They may feel helpless in managing their manifestations.

Both science and condition decide whether an individual will have anxiety. As it were, on edge conduct can be acquired, learned, or both. For instance, inquire about shows that on edge guardians are probably going to have on edge youngsters. Be that as it may, guardians may likewise display restless conduct. Assuming this is the case, they may impart that equivalent conduct in their kids. Having a stressful childhood can also expand an individual's odds of having anxiety. This is because anxiety turns into an approach to foresee risk and remain safe. Anxiety can likewise create because of uncertain trauma. Uncertain trauma may leave an individual in an elevated condition of physiological excitement. At the point when this is the situation, specific encounters can reactivate the old trauma. This is basic for individuals with posttraumatic stress (PTSD).

TYPES OF ANXIETY

Anxiety is at the base of numerous emotional well-being conditions, including alarm assaults and fears. It is regularly legitimately identified with different conditions, similar to fixations and impulses, PTSD, and depression. Notwithstanding summed up anxiety, the DSM-5 records the accompanying emotional wellness issues as anxiety issue:

- Separation anxiety: Can be portrayed by hesitance to venture out from home or be separated from guardians and anxiety when isolated from guardians.

- Selective mutism: Selective mutism implies not talking at all in just a few circumstances. This may cause issues with scholastic, work, or social achievement.

- Panic: The Panic issue is analyzed by repeating alarm assaults, including physical indications of anxiety.

- Specific fears: Phobias are dread encompassing a particular book or circumstance, which the individual keeps away from.

- Social anxiety: People with social anxiety feel dread or fear in social circumstances. The dread is frequently out of extent to the danger, and individuals with social anxiety may evade social circumstances.

- Agoraphobia: Agoraphobia can remember the dread of being for open or encased spaces, going out, and being in groups or utilizing accessible transportation.

- Medication/substance-instigated anxiety: This condition is analyzed by stress that is by all accounts legitimately brought about by presentation to specific substances, similar to caffeine or liquor. The anxiety could likewise be brought about by a drug.

ANXIETY IN CHILDREN

Youngsters, similar to grown-ups, can encounter anxiety. Be that as it may, kids may show unexpected side effects in comparison to adults. Realizing how to recognize anxiety in youngsters can help guardians or watchmen address it early. At that point, guardians may choose to discover a youngster therapist or analyst to help their kid figure out how to oversee it.

On the off chance that a youngster feels on edge more frequently and more strongly than most kids their age, they may have some anxiety. A kid who has anxiety may experience issues going to class. They may likewise keep away from social occasions or extracurricular exercises, similar to sports. A few children with anxiety are behind for their age in territories like making companions or being free. Anxiety in kids may show up as crying, sticking to guardians, or fits of rage.

Children with anxiety may show certain practices that copy fixations or impulses.

Ceaseless picking or pulling at skin or hair can be an on edge conduct. They may likewise give indications of partition anxiety. Indications of detachment anxiety incorporate sticking to guardians, crying, or declining to go to class or companion's homes. Youngsters can likewise encounter summed up anxiety and will be unable to recognize why they feel on edge. As youngsters enter pre-adulthood, they might be bound to create anxiety. Social anxiety frequently starts around age 13. Up to 25.1% of young people ages 13 to 18 might be influenced by an anxiety condition.

More established kids or youngsters may create nourishment related anxiety, which can prompt disarranged eating. Whenever left unchecked, this can cause genuine wellbeing confusions. Studies show that up to 91% of female teenagers have attempted to control their weight with nourishment. In the meantime, around 40% of female adolescents give indications of disarranged eating. A few specialists state that eating issues in guys are additionally expanding. While nourishment related anxiety can happen without anyone else, it regularly co-happens with other anxiety-related conditions, for example, fixations and impulses. Cluttered eating may likewise create in youngsters as a method for dealing with stress for handling anxiety, stress, or trauma.

EXAMPLES OF ANXIETY

Anxiety influences 18.1% of the grown-up populace in the United States; however, contemplates appear as not many as 36.9% of these individuals will get treatment for anxiety. One reason for this might be the absence of information about anxiety conditions. The disgrace that can accompany looking for help for psychological wellness could likewise add to this hole. Case instances of anxiety may help individuals recognize their indications and increment their familiarity with their prosperity; this can propel individuals to look for help for anxiety that is raising a ruckus in everyday life.

Anxiety can come in numerous structures and show in various ways. It very well may be helpful to understand how anxiety may influence you. Instances of various types of anxiety can encourage this procedure. Case models can show how assorted the side effects of anxiety can be and how stress can show up uniquely in contrast to an individual to an individual. Different auras and foundations may change how anxiety impacts somebody.

Individuals likewise handle their anxiety unexpectedly. Individuals may create hurtful ways of dealing with stress as a result of their anxiety, for instance. These methods for coping with stress frequently will, in general, worsen anxiety over the long haul. These models can help you distinguish what sort of anxiety you may have and help you realize what you can do to address it.

CASE EXAMPLES OF ANXIETY

- **Alcohol Abuse and Anxiety:** Hayat, 23, encounters extreme fits of anxiety. These happen when she believes she has fizzled at an assignment or irritated somebody. Now and then they happen when she gets analysis. She starts to experience difficulty breathing, becomes sweat-soaked, and may break out in hives. Her brain turns out to be centered around the offence she has submitted. She may cry; however, she smothers the tears and averts purge. She drinks enormous amounts of liquor to help numb herself to these emotions.

In some cases, she misses work for quite a long time. This promotes her anxiety, as she has a little salary. She starts looking for treatment for liquor compulsion. Her therapist sees that anxiety is by all accounts the more profound issue. In therapy, Hayat learns more beneficial approaches to adapt to her anxiety.

- **Social Anxiety:** Benji, 45, is well known at work and extremely skilled. Be that as it may, he feels exceptionally on edge at whatever point he is out in the open. He is particularly on edge around swarms. He races home every night, bolts his entryway, and peruses in bed. When he is distant from everyone else with the loft, he has a sense of safety. He can't distinguish the reason for his anxiety. Be that as it may, in therapy, he finds a lot of subdued outrage. This starts to clarify his dread of being out in the open. Individuals trigger his wrath, which he has kept away from for quite a long time.

- **"People-Pleasing" Anxiety:** Anna, 26, comes to therapy on account of extreme anxiety. Anna has not encountered a fit of anxiety. Be that as it may, she is frequently anxious, stressed, stressed, and experiences difficulty staying asleep from sundown to sunset. Anna starts going to therapy. She finds that she has stifled some significant sentiments. Albeit some portion of her needs to wed her life partner, another piece of herself isn't infatuated with him. Discovering this interior clash from the start increases Anna's anxiety. She currently needs to confront something she hasn't required a face. Verifiably, Anna has been an accommodating person. It's hard for her to state "no" inspired by a paranoid fear of offending others and then feeling her blame. Anna picks up mindfulness about this. She starts unburdening her since quite a while ago harboured blame. Anna begins feeling less anxiety once again enabling others to feel torment. Anna hasn't yet chosen what she will do about getting hitched. However, she presently feels less anxiety, as she is never again stifling her irresoluteness. She has more certainty about imparting how she truly feels.

HOW TO GET HELP FOR ANXIETY

Anxiety can meddle with relationships, rest, dietary patterns, work, school, and leisure activities. It is likewise one of the most widely recognized reasons individuals look for therapy. Powerful therapy can diminish or take out indications that accompany anxiety in a genuinely brief time. Although individuals will most likely be unable to pinpoint the reason for their anxiety, therapy can help them discover it. Therapists frequently help individuals take a shot at numerous anxiety-related concerns.

It can take some time for an individual with anxiety to open up to a therapist. It might require some investment for them to feel they can confide in the therapeutic relationship and procedure. In any case, adhering to a solid therapy plan can yield incredible achievement. There are many proof-based strategies for treating anxiety. You and your therapist can discover one that works best for you.

WHEN TO GET HELP FOR ANXIETY

If you think you have anxiety, there will never be a terrible time to connect for help. The following are a few signs; it may be an ideal opportunity to look for proficient guidance for anxiety:

- You have contemplations that vibe startling or crazy

- Anxiety is contrarily affecting relationships you care about

- You feel like you can't be out in the open or around others.

- You are experiencing difficulty dozing.

- Anxiety makes it difficult to do everyday undertakings like eating, cleaning, getting down to business, or youngster care.

- You are pondering harming yourself.

<u>KINDS OF THERAPY FOR ANXIETY</u>

The kind of therapy regularly utilized for treating anxiety is psychological behavioral therapy (CBT). Numerous investigations have demonstrated it is viable. CBT works by retraining how individuals thoroughly consider introduction. For instance, a therapist may teach an individual who is restless about going out to go on short errands. As the individual in therapy turns out to be progressively agreeable, they may go out for longer measures of time. In the long run, they may feel progressively good doing as such.

Although CBT is utilized frequently, numerous types of therapy are appropriate to take a shot at anxiety. Therapy doesn't just regard the manifestations of anxiety as prescription does. Instead, it tends to the wellspring of the anxiety. Therapy's self-intelligent procedure helps individuals understand, unwind, and change anxiety. Individuals in treatment for anxiety figure out how to self-relieve. If anxiety erupts once more, having sound adapting abilities can be vital.

Different kinds of therapy that are regularly used to treat anxiety include:

- Biofeedback: This kind of therapy utilizes, in essence, attention to treat anxiety. It can help individuals understand how they respond to stress physically.

- Mindfulness-based cognitive therapy (MBCT): MBCT brings care practices to subjective social therapy. It has been appeared to diminish anxiety by helping individuals increment their self-mindfulness in therapy.

- Dialectical behavioral therapy (DBT): This kind of therapy is frequently utilized for "hard to treat" conditions. It might help individuals with extreme anxiety balance out, investigate their anxiety, improve their satisfaction, and keep up a feeling of prosperity.

- Psychodynamic therapy: Psychodynamic therapy can help individuals with anxiety by pointing out their very own idea examples and propensities. It might likewise energize diving into the subliminal to get to the underlying driver of the anxiety.

- Eye development desensitization resolution (EMDR): EMDR utilizes eye development methods to help individuals get too troublesome recollections and can be helpful with treating anxiety.

- Hakomi Experiential Therapy: Using the act of care, an individual with anxiety will work with a prepared therapist to search internally. They will achieve deceptions themselves into awareness and address them. The therapist may help the individual substitute those thoughts with increasingly useful ones. This kind of therapy can be physical. This implies if the individual in therapy assents, contact might be utilized to pass on help and support.

- Hypnotherapy: Hypnotherapy can be utilized to treat fears and anxiety. It can help individuals accomplish self-investigation and understanding by moving beyond the cognizant idea.

AUGMENTING EFFECTIVENESS OF THERAPY FOR ANXIETY

Methods of therapy are various ways a kind of therapy can be led. It can incorporate what number of individuals are in therapy with you and how you get treatment. As anxiety can display its own arrangement of difficulties, specific methods of therapy might be pretty much compelling for an individual with anxiety than somebody with another condition.

Once in a while, impediments keep individuals from finding support for anxiety. An individual with social anxiety may feel nervous about gathering a therapist face to face or calling them on the telephone. Agoraphobia or other explicit fears can likewise make individuals hesitant to go out or drive in a vehicle. These exercises are regularly fundamental for getting to therapy. For this situation, finding a therapist who can meet you in your home can be helpful. Or then again, you may decide to talk with a separation therapist on the web or the telephone.

A few people with anxiety may think that its helpful to talk with others with comparative encounters. These individuals could profit by bunch therapy for anxiety. In a gathering therapy session, individuals can talk about and find out about their anxiety together, drove by an authorized therapist. Not exclusively can the gathering therapy experience be approving for some individuals; it can likewise help them practice abilities they can use to diminish anxiety with other gathering individuals.

PRESCRIPTION FOR ANXIETY

Psychotropic meds for anxiety are intended to treat the side effects of stress and enable an individual to capacity and feel good. Nonetheless, they can't address hidden passionate and mental reasons for anxiety or help individuals figure out how to adapt to future situations that could expedite an on-edge reaction. Basic drugs for anxiety incorporate antidepressants, for example, Celexa, Lexapro, Prozac, and Zoloft, and against anxiety prescriptions like Ativan, Xanax, and Klonopin. Undesirable symptoms are normal, and every individual will unexpectedly react to the drug. It is critical to follow changes in disposition, conduct, and different manifestations to locate the correct medicine. For somebody who is deadened by anxiety or has extraordinary frenzy, drug might be fundamental to driving a satisfying life.

WAY OF LIFE CHANGES THAT CAN REDUCE ANXIETY

Therapy can be a significant piece of working through any anxiety you have. Notwithstanding treatment, individual propensities may likewise help diminish your stress. It very well may be beneficial to consider aspects of your life where you can feel less restless. Once in a while, an individual in therapy may even work with their therapist to make an arrangement that incorporates a portion of these ways of life changes. Remember that a portion of this way of life changes may not be for everybody.

A large number of this way of life changes are self-care propensities and include:

- Keeping a diary

- Meditation

- Practising care

- Exercise

- Yoga

- Getting enough rest

- Cutting out or diminishing admission of energizers like caffeine

<u>HELP IS HERE</u>

Anxiety can feel overpowering. Untreated, it might develop progressively extreme and can prompt disengagement, depression, and contemplations of suicide. If you feel adversely affected by anxiety, you can discover a therapist to work with.

CHAPTER SEVEN

THE KEY ROLE YOUR NERVOUS SYSTEM PLAYS IN TRAUMA RECOVERY

If you somehow managed to go to an expert preparing on trauma, the educator would almost certainly reference the nervous system and its window of resistance. As of late, trauma analysts and therapists have built up a more profound understanding of the nervous system's job in directing excessive stress, and have adapted a few methods for controlling this system.

You have likely known about the fight-or-flight reaction, which portrays our drive to protect ourselves or run until we arrive at wellbeing. This is a piece of the window-of-resilience model, yet it's not exactly the entire picture. We should begin with understanding a managed nervous system.

A directed nervous system encounters stress and quieting reaction over a given day. Maybe you are driving and somebody brakes startlingly in front of you;

when your nervous system is managed you will feel some stress, yet once your body has a sense of security and you can act in a manner to guarantee your wellbeing (i.e., press your very own brakes), your system will quiet back to gauge. Dr Dan Siegel of UCLA instituted the expression "window of resistance" to portray this space where we can manage ourselves without a lot of exertion.

Make sense? You've likely felt a portion of these changes in your system today—racing to get someplace and loosening up when you land on schedule, for instance. Next, we'll investigate what occurs the nervous system when a traumatic encounter enters the image.

Trauma pushes the actuation of the nervous system past its capacity to self-direct. At the point when a stressful encounter pushes the system past its breaking points, it can get stuck "on." When an order is overstimulated like this, we can encounter anxiety, alarm, outrage, hyperactivity, and eagerness. This is the fight-or-flight mode; your body is initiated and prepared to move.

Some nervous systems will remain here, while others will plunge beneath the typical range and get stuck on "off." Below the window of resistance, we see side effects of depression, exhaustion, disconnection, and dormancy. Systems can stall out above or underneath the line for delayed timeframes, or they can waver between the two.

How might you release the traumatic stress and progress once more into the window of the managed nervous system? Here are a couple of tips:

1. Look for safe relationships. Being with somebody who is sheltered and alleviating will help your nervous system settle and make a protected space for you to interface and offer your experience. We are social creatures, and we mend in a relationship, so on the off chance that you wind up disconnecting or pulling endlessly from social contact, consider instead searching out individuals who feel steady.

2. Practice careful relaxing. This trauma reaction is associated with the brain stem (essential physiological guideline) and the limbic (enthusiastic) brain. Rehearsing mindful breathing helps interface a fundamental physiological procedure (breathing) with your prefrontal cortex (thinking brain), which helps coordinate and move our neurological state. To put that all the more essentially: breathing has a HUGE ability

to quiet the brain and control the nervous system.

3. Discover a therapist who understands trauma and can help you become acquainted with the propensities for your nervous system. Perceiving when you are outside of your window of resilience and building individual techniques to relieve or animate your system is critical to managing in a progressing way. For specific individuals, sitting still is quieting; for other people,

development brings more harmony. Discover somebody who can bolster you as you investigate what works best for you.

There are numerous one of a kind and sound ways you can figure out how to help your nervous system and bring it over into its window of resistance when something stressful happens. Making a supportive group of people that incorporates a prepared trauma therapist is a helpful method to assemble your capacity to mend and recoup from traumatic encounters. At the point when you figure out how to function with your nervous system, you may even develop a more extensive window of resistance, which can enable you to move about the world inclination more grounded and associated with others.

EYE MOVEMENT DESENSITIZATION AND REPROCESSING THERAPY (EMDR)

Eye movement desensitization and reprocessing (EMDR), created by Dr. Francine Shapiro, is an exploration bolstered, integrative psychotherapy approach intended to treat manifestations of trauma and posttraumatic stress. EMDR sessions pursue a particular arrangement of stages, and experts utilize reciprocal stimulation, for example, eye movements, to help the customer process uncertain recollections from unfriendly encounters. EMDR can be used to address any number of concerns, and it is perfect with different sorts of therapy.

THE THEORY BEHIND EMDR THERAPY

The versatile data processing (AIP) model—the hypothetical structure for EMDR therapy—clarifies that a few recollections related to unfavorable beneficial encounters may stay unprocessed because of the significant level of unsettling influence experienced at the hour of the occasion. The put-away memory might be connected to feelings, pessimistic insights, and physical sensations experienced during the occasion, and the unprocessed mind can influence how an individual reacts to, resulting in comparable unfavorable encounters. Through EMDR therapy, these divided recollections can be reprocessed, so they become progressively intelligible and less problematic.

<u>EMDR'S EFFECTIVENESS</u>

EMDR has been acknowledged as a compelling type of treatment by a few significant wellbeing associations, including the World Health Organization, the American Psychiatric Association, and the Department of Defense. Studies demonstrate that it is conceivable to lighten distressing side effects more quickly with EMDR than with talk therapy alone. PTSD was wiped out for 100% of individuals who had encountered a solitary traumatic occasion and for 77% who had faced various traumas following six 50-minute sessions. Since talking about the subtleties of a traumatic encounter isn't required in EMDR sessions, the uneasiness related to standing up to and uncovering those subtleties might be lightened.

<u>HOW ARE EMDR THERAPY SESSIONS?</u>

Although EMDR was initially intended to treat posttraumatic stress, it very well may be utilized to address other unfavorable beneficial encounters or negative convictions. In the customary course of therapy, the advisor and the individual in therapy may recognize a distressing occasion or contrary belief that would profit by EMDR. The expert will spend in any event one therapy session portraying EMDR and setting up the individual for the process, and explicit EMDR sessions will be planned.

EMDR therapy is an eight-stage approach that distinguishes and processes recollections of negative and traumatic occasions that add to display issues. After the individual in treatment quickly gets to an uncertain memory, the person will concentrate on the outer stimulus conveyed by the therapist. These signals can incorporate eye movement, taps, or tones. During each arrangement of reciprocal stimulus, or double consideration, new affiliations develop as bits of knowledge, different recollections, and new feelings. After each set, the customer quickly reports what grew in awareness, and the following focal point of consideration is distinguished for processing. The processing focuses during EMDR therapy incorporate past occasions, current triggers, and future needs. The eight periods of EMDR therapy include:

1. History taking: The therapist and customer audit past occasions, current concerns and future needs, and distinguish target occasions for processing.

2. Preparation: To get ready for adapting to any distress that may emerge during the desensitization stage, the individual in therapy chooses a sheltered spot picture that can give adjustment and self-control varying.

3. Assessment: With the distressing occasion as a primary concern, the customer's

negative convictions about himself or herself are recorded, assessed, and estimated. Interestingly, an alluring definite conviction is chosen, and this conviction is estimated to decide how obvious it feels to the customer. Physical manifestations are also recorded.

4. Desensitization: Bilateral stimulation, like eye movements, tones, or taps, are utilized to reprocess the distressing occasion. The therapist will occasionally break to monitor the customer's degree of unsettling influence.

5. Installation: The chose positive perception is the objective of the two-sided stimulation in this stage. The therapist will check in

occasionally to perceive how obvious the ideal conviction feels to the customer.

6. Body output: Any remaining physical pressure or distress demonstrates that the occasion isn't completely processed, and the two-sided stimulation proceeds, if vital.

7. Closure: This stage will happen toward the finish of a session, paying little mind to whether the memory is completely processed. A total grouping of EMDR therapy can take a few sessions, and it is essential to arrive at adjustment before the session closes. The conclusion can incorporate guided symbolism or discourse of the session.

8. Reevaluation: The following session starts here to assess and gauge the degree of aggravation and the precision of the focused on positive conviction. If the objective stays uncertain, the session will continue with desensitization, stage 4.

The two critical components of EMDR therapy are recognized as the conviction that eye movements improve the adequacy of remedial treatment through the advancement of physiological and neurological changes and that these progressions help the customer in healing and recuperating from the negative recollections. Research has additionally demonstrated that eye movement is a physiological strategy for inner desensitization to the passionate response to the memory.

TREATING TRAUMA: WHY EMDR MIGHT BE RIGHT FOR YOU

The primary inquiry an individual who is seeking help for trauma regularly asks is, "Will I ever show signs of improvement?" It is normal to feel sad in the wake of encountering a traumatic occasion. Trauma influences how the brain capacities. It can physically change the brain and make individuals feel that they are not themselves anymore. Exercises that were once basic and programmed become troublesome or feel downright incomprehensible. Luckily, the alternatives for the treatment of trauma are powerful. There are a few choices with regards to picking a methodology of trauma treatment. Having information about every method can help an individual to settle on an educated decision while choosing the course of treatment that is directly for the person in question.

Eye movement desensitization and reprocessing (EMDR) is one powerful technique for treating trauma. The name of this mediation is a significant piece; simply observing or hearing it can make an individual vibe overpowered and befuddled. It is, as a general rule, a genuinely essential intercession that tends to the numerous impacts of trauma, including negative convictions about the self, (for example, "I am undependable" or "I am awful") that generally emerge, the tangible viewpoint, including pictures and body sensations identified with the trauma, just as feelings. As indicated by the EMDR Institute, Inc., a few investigations have been directed to test the viability of EMDR, and the information shows that a dominant part of individuals experiences a decrease in their trauma-related side effects after treatment. One such investigation, directed via Carlson et al. (1998), found that 77.7% of veterans who had encountered different traumatic occasions had an end of posttraumatic stress (PTSD) manifestations in the wake of partaking in 12 sessions of EMDR. Another analysis, directed by Arabia et al. (2011), found that individuals who had encountered a dangerous medical problem identified with cardiovascular issues had a decrease in side effects identified with PTSD, depression, and nervousness.

OVERVIEW OF EMDR TREATMENT

There are eight stages in EMDR treatment. Francine Shapiro, who built up this therapeutic method, expresses that understand that to what extent an individual must spend in each step will be distinctive for every person.

The stages include:

1. Getting a history

2. Preparing an individual for the trauma work through building adapting aptitudes

3. Determining the particular segments of the primary trauma that will be reprocessed

4. Desensitization

5. Installing a positive conviction about the self when reviewing the trauma

6. Checking in with the body for any leftover trauma (body filter)

7. Closing of the session

8. Reevaluation during the following session to check whether any new

data has come up or changes have occurred between sessions

THE ROLE OF DUAL ATTENTION STIMULUS

What a great many people find captivating or even bizarre about EMDR is what is called double consideration stimulus, which is used during the desensitization, establishment, and body filter periods of EMDR. This includes either moving the eyes to and fro, tapping on one side of the body, and then the other (i.e., left hand and then right hand), or utilizing sounds in substituting ears.

The double consideration appears to do a couple of things: helps the brain to work through beforehand troublesome material, makes reviewing memory simpler, and has a quieting impact. It is obscure why the double consideration has this impact; however, a few investigations bolster its adequacy.

Double consideration can likewise help an individual to keep the consideration in the present while enabling the brain to go to the past, which can help to diminish the potential for hyperarousal, which could impede treatment. It is additionally thought to help with moving data through the brain, so it very well may be documented accurately.

HOW EMDR HELPS THE BRAIN

Another approach to see the EMDR process and how it helps to envision that your brain and its memory systems are a system of streams and waterways. At the point when a traumatic occasion occurs, it is practically similar to a beaver dam that has been built someplace inside the system, which can send the whole system into alarm mode. The water gets supported up and floods, which can influence territories that don't appear to be associated with the system with the square.

On account of trauma, it is the feeling, recollections, body sensations, musings, and convictions that are flooding and not getting where they have to go. EMDR's principle objective is to address and evacuate the beaver dam, or square, with the goal that the brain can process. Expelling squares helps the brain to take advantage of its capacity to recuperate itself.

IS IT RIGHT FOR YOU?

Whenever keen on taking an interest in EMDR therapy, ensure that a legitimate source prepared the therapist you pick. EMDR is a well-looked into and compelling treatment for trauma on any level, regardless of how little or large.

3 STEPS TO HEALING TRAUMA THAT EVERYONE SHOULD KNOW

The vast majority have had a traumatic encounter or something to that effect. While a large number of us figure out how to adapt and be flexible even with trauma, others may become overpowering.

Trauma is a staggering encounter, and it is our experience and response, more than the occasion itself, that characterizes trauma. The Diagnostic and Statistical Manual of Mental Disorders criteria for posttraumatic stress (PTSD) are explicit and include being presented to something that undermines life;

be that as it may, various individuals have a scope of reactions to comparable circumstances. What may feel commonplace to you could be traumatic to me, and the other way around. No judgment here—we are altogether wired unexpectedly.

The following are three straightforward advances that can help anybody confronting a staggering beneficial encounter—be it a cataclysmic event, loss of a friend or family member, an encounter of savagery, or an oppressive past.

When we've experienced a trauma, how would we get past it?

1. Seek safety. The initial phase intending to trauma is to make

safety, on various levels. Physically, discover a spot to ground yourself and feel shielded from hurt. At that point, search for approaches to effectively sustain yourself. Think about a feathered creature flying along and running into a glass window. What does that feathered creature need—maybe a little shoebox with some water and nourishment, and cherishing hands and eyes to look out for it? On an enthusiastic level, seek out those individuals throughout your life who can watch out for you as you would that feathered creature, who offer love, backing, mindful, and understanding. If you have a system of loved ones, approach them. There are likewise individuals and associations out there to help, serve, and bolster you. Additionally, seek support on an otherworldly level. Associating with a higher power or more profound insight that impacts you can be a redeeming quality. Many inclines toward nature. Find what mitigates your spirit.

2. Process. When you feel more grounded, contained, and safe (and you think READY for this progression), you can start to process

the pieces of the experience that are still with you. Look to your body and discover the development that helps you connect with yourself and your sentiments. Locate a decent therapist or gathering wherein you can talk straightforwardly and genuinely. As you process, you'll keep on creating adapting abilities and qualities and expand upon the safety and control you've made.

3. Examine. At the point when the more significant part of your processing is finished, life goes on. The objective isn't to overlook the traumatic experience yet to

determine the passionate charge it holds in the present. Take a gander at any learning or development that has originated from this experience. What bits of knowledge have you picked up? Cause a note to yourself of any positive things you to have discovered that you can convey forward.

At the point when we process one life occasion thoroughly, we may find more there—different encounters or things we have found out about ourselves that merit consideration and healing. At this point, ideally, you have great relationships and supports you can incline toward to proceed with your healing voyage carefully, with sympathy for yourself and with the information that endeavors put toward healing will be helpful for you

THE TRAUMA OF WORKPLACE STRESS: HOW THERAPY CAN HELP

A large portion of us experience work stress, however, can an excessive number of duties, ridiculous desires, and character clashes at work lead to an encounter of trauma victimization after some time?

In my long periods of private psychotherapy practice, I've seen a few situations where people experience signs like posttraumatic stress because of work issues. First and foremost, I discovered this somewhat odd. I pondered: could negative work encounters truly lead to responses like trauma encounters, similar to war or rape? Of late, in discussions with associates, I've found this is genuinely normal, especially in specific callings.

HOW YOUR WORK ENVIRONMENT CAN LEAVE YOU FEELING VICTIMIZED

Accepting I talked with Arkansas proficient advocate, who is an appointed clergyman who left the service to turn into a therapist. She has some expertise in advising ministers and their families and said that feeling victimized and traumatized by their workplace is moderately regular among individuals from the ministry. She may clarify that the demands and desires for present-day service set ministers up for personal disappointment and enthusiastic trauma.

"The standards in service are defective. A hundred years prior, ministers had four occupations: wed, cover, sanctify through water, and lecture on Sunday. Today, clergymen are relied upon to be marriage therapists and misery counselors, authoritative pioneers, offices and staff directors, showcasing organizers, network relations pros, bloggers, persuasive orator, profound instructors, sales reps (expanding participation and giving), spending chiefs, visit the wiped out, be a companion, and serve on territorial panels! It's unreasonable. It sets everybody up for dissatisfaction."

These encounters are like what's going on in privately owned businesses as of late, especially since the financial accident of 2008. Organizations have laid-off individuals and expect individuals who stay to accomplish more work for less pay. New execution measures are including weight, and representatives are micromanaged. Among the EAP (Employee Assistance Program) referrals I find in my office, stress identified with new and ridiculous work execution desires positions at the highest priority on the rundown.

The individuals who see me for help with business-related stress have grumblings that are like what the minister sees among church: a sleeping disorder, peevishness, mind-set swings, outrage, sentiments of frustration and thwarted expectation about their vocation and manager, disarray concerning why they can't satisfy the needs put on them, misery, uneasiness and dread, weakness, muscle pressure, family issues, sentiments of disconnection, ineffectual adapting, and substance misuse. It's a considerable rundown! Work stress is a significant issue in America.

Vast numbers of us know about trauma responses after significant fiascoes. Yet, not many of us understand that a workplace portrayed by unreasonable demands, character clashes, and constrained available time for recreation can, in the long run, make an encounter of victimization.

3 WAYS COGNITIVE BEHAVIORAL THERAPY CAN HELP

Cognitive Behavioral Therapy (CBT) helps people move from seeing themselves as having little command over their conditions to getting enabled to either change outside weights or figure out how to adapt to and unexpectedly identify with them. With training, CBT strategies can help decrease stress and nervousness, improve the state of mind, and increment certainty.

CBT treatment has helped pastors diminish the experience of stress and trauma brought about by the difficulties of their calling. These equivalent procedures can likewise help the vast majority mend from different traumatic and sincerely troublesome circumstances. CBT lessens distress and helps to reestablish passionate parity. Here are three methods of intellectual conduct therapy to use in your own life.

1. Learn to recognize the musings that expansion your nervousness and your self-question. A vast, more

significant part of people who come to see me for nervousness therapy is very astounded when I notice that their contemplations are likely causing their uneasiness. The vast majority accept nervousness is something that transpires, something over which they have no control. In any case, truth be told, how we converse with ourselves about the circumstances we face has a lot to do with how we feel. For instance, if a pastor reveals to herself that since her congregation isn't developing, she isn't a successful pioneer and has bombed God, she is probably going to feel genuinely annoyed and accept that she isn't equipped for developing the congregation. By rehashing self-overcoming musings in her mind, her self-regard dissolves. In the long run, she may quit any pretense of attempting through and through and become discouraged. This is the stunt trauma plays on us: it discloses to us that something isn't right with us and that we are helpless; however, more often than not, our musings are not valid.

2. Dispute the idea. When you've distinguished the nervousness creating or self-crushing idea, it's an

excellent opportunity to question it. Here's a model: "On the off chance that I don't develop the congregation, I'll get terminated." Let's examine if that contemplation is valid. In many divisions, terminating a minister requires exertion. To begin with, the administration of the congregation needs to cast a ballot that they have lost trust in the minister. At that point, they need to carry the issue to a congregational vote. As a rule, a national middle person gets included to help settle the contention and improve the representative/manager connection between the congregation and the minister. So the idea, "On the off chance that I don't develop the congregation, I'll get terminated" isn't valid. What's considerably more liable to happen is that if the congregation isn't developing and pioneers are disappointed, a discussion will occur regarding for what reason that is going on. And ideally, that discussion will prompt arrangements. Notice your very own contemplations and question them. Is it true that they are valid? How would you know without a doubt? What are some alternative clarifications that may be all the more obvious?

3. Learn to relax. The third CBT system that the minister utilizes is unraveling preparing. At the point when we figure out how to loosen up the pressure in our muscles and lessen the speed of our considerations, our brains work better. They see things all the more unmistakably. Gen. Colin Powell has a standard. He lets himself know, "It isn't as awful as you might suspect. It will glance better toward the beginning of the day." That's incomplete because when our brains

are refreshed, we see circumstances unexpectedly. Unwinding preparing can instruct you to rest your brain. I expect that one day, we will all things considered to figure out how to be reasonable about our demands and desires for individuals and be kinder to each other. Up to that point, on the off chance that you end up feeling victimized, exorbitantly forced, or question your value or capacities, attempt CBT. It truly can help!